Floraopathy™
The Art and Science of Vibrational Healing with Essential Oils

Dr. Constance Santego

Maximillian Enterprises
Kelowna, BC

Floraopathy™: The Art and Science of Vibrational Healing with Essential Oils

Copyright © 2024 by Constance Santego.

Copy Editor & Interior Design: Constance Santego
Book Layout: ©2017 BookDesignTemplates.com

Ordering Information:
Quantity sales. Special discounts are available on quantity purchases by corporations, associations, and others. Contact the "Special Sales Department" at the address below for details.

Trade Paperback ISBN: 978-1-990062-41-4
eBook ISBN 978-1-990062-42-1
Created and published In Canada. Printed and bound in the United States of America

First Edition
Published by Maximillian Enterprises
Kelowna, BC
Canada
www.constancesantego.ca

ALSO BY DR. CONSTANCE SANTEGO

FICTION
The Nine Spiritual Gifts Series:
Journey of a Soul – (Vol 1 Michael)
Language of a Soul – (Vol 2 Gabriel)
Prophecy of a Soul – (Vol 3 Bath Kol)
Healing of a Soul – (Vol 4 Raphael)
Miracles of a Soul – (Vol 5 Hamied)
Knowledge of a Soul – (Vol 6 Raziel)

NONFICTION
The Intuitive Life, The Gift of Prophecy, Third Edition
Fairy Tales, Dreams and Reality… Where Are You On Your Path? Second Edition
Your Persona… The Mask You Wear
Angelic Lifestyle, A Vibrant Lifestyle
Angelic Lifestyle 42-Day Energy Cleanse
Archangel Michael's Soul Retrieval Guide
Tesla and the Future of Energy Medicine
Scaling Beyond 6 Figures: *Strategies for Health & Wellness Professionals*
Beyond the Mind: *Harnessing the Power of Astral Projection for Creative Awakening*
Bend, Don't Break: *Finding Your Way Back to Abundance*
Ring Therapy: *A Guide to Healing and Balance*
Ring Therapy Pocket Guide

SECRETS OF A HEALER, SERIES:
Magic Of Aromatherapy (Vol I)
Magic Of Reflexology (Vol II)
Magic Of The Gifts (Vol III)
Magic Of Muscle Testing (Vol IV)
Magic Of Iridology (Vol V)
Magic Of Massage (Vol VI)
Magic Of Hypnotherapy (Vol VII)
Magic Of Reiki (Vol VIII)
Magic Of Advanced Aromatherapy (Vol IX)
Magic Of Esthetics (Vol X)
Reiki Master's Manual (Vol XI)

ADULT COLORING JOURNALS

SERIES - ZEN COLORING:
Quantum Energy and Mindful Living Journal (Vol 1)
Reiki Energy Journal (Vol 2)
Nine Spiritual Gifts Journal (Vol 3)
I Forgive Journal (Vol 4)

SERIES - COLORING PROSPERITY:
Genie-Inspired Mandalas and Wealth Journal (Vol 1)
Entrepreneurial Mindset Reboot (Vol 2)

SERIES - HARMONIC MIND CODE:
Harmonic Mind Code Coloring Journal (Vol 1)

FOR CHILDREN
I am Big Tonight. I Don't Need the Light!

COOKBOOK
My Favorite Recipes, with a Hint of Giggle

Dedication to
Doug and Sue Thompson and Evelen Mulders

Shift Happens…Create Magic!

—Dr. Constance Santego

Preface

Welcome to Floraopathy™: The Art and Science of Vibrational Healing with Essential Oils

In an age where holistic health practices are increasingly sought after, this book introduces a unique and transformative approach to healing through Floraopathy. Integrating the timeless wisdom of vibrational energy healing with the therapeutic power of essential oils, Floraopathy offers a comprehensive guide to achieving balance and wellness.

Understanding Floraopathy

Floraopathy is more than just a method of treatment; it is an art form rooted in the science of vibrational healing. By harnessing the natural vibrational frequencies of essential oils, Floraopathy aims to restore harmony within the body's energetic systems. This practice is built on the principle that each plant possesses a distinct vibrational energy that can be used to heal and balance various physical, emotional, and spiritual conditions.

The Foundation of Vibrational Healing

Vibrational healing acknowledges that every being and object in the universe vibrates at its own unique frequency. When the body's natural frequencies are disrupted, it can lead to imbalance and illness. With their potent and specific vibrational qualities, essential oils can help realign these frequencies, promoting healing and well-being.

The Power of Essential Oils

Essential oils are the lifeblood of plants, carrying their healing properties and vibrational energy. These oils have been used for centuries in various cultures for their therapeutic benefits. In Floraopathy, we explore how these oils can be utilized for their biochemical effects and their ability to influence the body's energy fields.

Purpose of This Book

This book serves as a practical and insightful guide for anyone interested in exploring the healing potential of Floraopathy. Whether you are a seasoned practitioner or new to the world of holistic health, this book provides valuable information on how to incorporate vibrational healing with essential oils into your daily life.

What You Will Learn

- **Foundational Principles:** Understand the basics of vibrational healing and the role of essential oils in this practice.
- **Properties of Essential Oils**: Discover the unique vibrational qualities of various essential oils and their specific healing properties.
- **Practical Applications:** Learn how to create and use Floraopathy blends to address different health conditions and support overall wellness.
- Case Studies and Examples: Explore real-life examples and case studies that illustrate the effectiveness of Floraopathy.
- **Integration with Other Practices:** Find out how to combine Floraopathy with other holistic health practices for enhanced healing.

How to Use This Book

This book offers a glimpse into the world of Floraopathy™, providing an introduction to its principles and practices. It lays the foundation for understanding the vibrational properties of essential oils and how they can be used to enhance your health and well-being. Consider this book as a starting point, inspiring you to delve deeper into Floraopathy™ through further study and practice. It's an essential read for anyone interested in exploring the transformative power of essential oils and holistic healing.

Important Notice on Liability and Consulting a Doctor

Disclaimer

The information provided in this book is intended for educational purposes only and should not be considered medical advice. The practices and suggestions described herein are based on traditional knowledge and contemporary applications. They are not intended to diagnose, treat, cure, or prevent any disease.

Liability

The author and publisher of this book assume no responsibility for any adverse effects, injuries, or damages that may result from the use or misuse of the information contained herein. Readers are strongly advised to use their own judgment and discretion when applying the practices discussed in this book.

Consulting a Doctor

Consulting with a qualified healthcare provider is crucial before beginning any new health regimen, incorporating supplements, or using alternative healing practices such as those described in this book. This is especially important for individuals with pre-existing health conditions, those who are pregnant or breastfeeding, and those currently taking medications. Your healthcare provider can offer personalized advice and ensure that any new practices are safe and appropriate for your specific health needs. They can also provide guidance on proper dosages and monitor for potential interactions with other treatments you may be undergoing.

Safety First

While traditional practices offer valuable insights into health and wellness, modern medical guidance is essential to ensure your safety and well-being. Always prioritize professional medical advice and support when considering changes to your health routine.

By consulting with your healthcare provider and using this book as a supplementary resource, you can make informed decisions that contribute to your overall health and well-being.

Dr. Constance Santego

Contents

"Nature itself is the
best physician."

— Hippocrates

Floraopathy™

The Art and Science of Vibrational Healing with Essential Oils

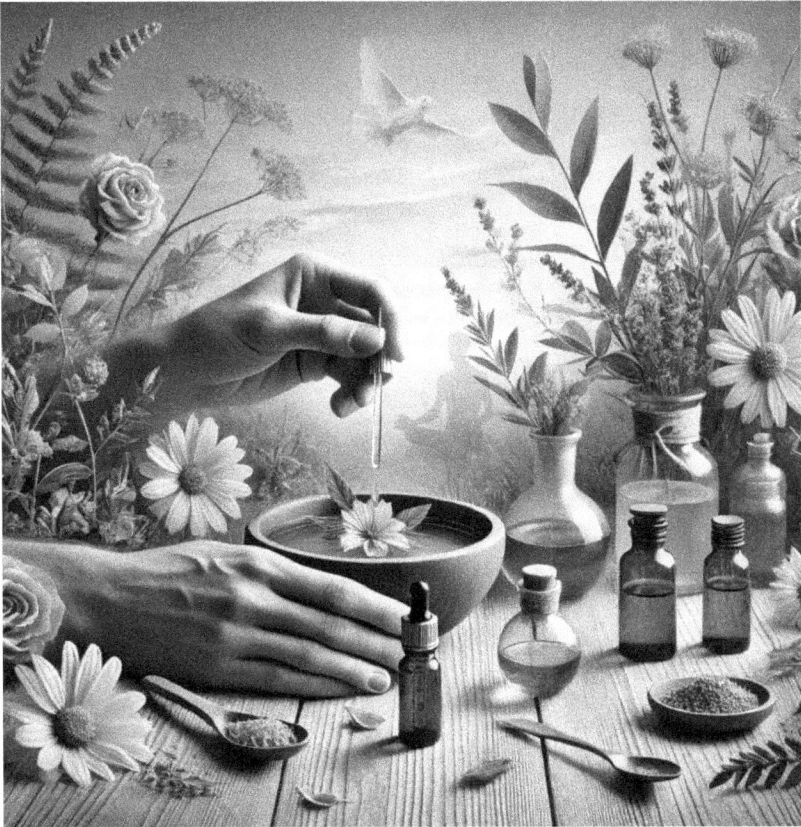

Dr. Constance Santego

CHAPTER 1: INTRODUCTION

What is Floraopathy™?

Floraopathy™ is a unique and innovative approach to vibrational energy healing that utilizes the therapeutic properties of essential oils. This method involves a specialized blending technique of plant steam-distilled essential oils to create personalized treatments aimed at harmonizing the body, mind, and soul. Practitioners of Floraopathy™ use various blends, including therapeutic cross-referencing blends, bath blends, spritzers, and EMP (Emotional, Mental, Physical) blends, to address and balance different aspects of a person's well-being.

Definition and Overview

Floraopathy™ combines principles from aromatherapy, homeopathy, and flower essences. Like homeopathy, it embraces the concept of potentized doses, and similar to flower essences and Bach remedies, it addresses the spiritual causes of symptoms. The distinguishing factor of Floraopathy™ lies in its unique blend selection process, the specific products used, and the method of combination. Essential oils have been utilized for centuries for their healing properties, and Floraopathy™ brings a new dimension by integrating these oils into a comprehensive system that targets emotional, spiritual, mental, and physical health.

Historical Background and Development

The word "Floraopathy™" is derived from "flora," referring to the plant life occurring in a particular region, and "opathy," a suffix derived from the Greek word "pathos," meaning suffering or disease. The practice of Floraopathy™ combines ancient wisdom with modern scientific understanding of essential oils and their effects on the human body.

The roots of Floraopathy™ can be traced back to the holistic health traditions of aromatherapy and homeopathy, which have long recognized the healing potential of plants. Over the years, practitioners have refined the techniques and methods of using essential oils to create personalized treatments that cater to the specific needs of individuals. The development of Floraopathy™ represents the culmination of these efforts, offering a structured and practical approach to holistic healing.

In this book, we will explore the fundamental principles of Floraopathy™, the properties of various essential oils, and practical applications for integrating this powerful healing method into your daily life. Whether you are new to vibrational healing or looking to deepen your understanding, this guide provides valuable insights and tools to enhance your well-being through the art and science of Floraopathy™.

Welcome to the world of Floraopathy™, where ancient traditions meet modern science to create a holistic approach to health and wellness.

Floraopathy™ Prerequisites and Required Materials

To fully appreciate and practice Floraopathy™, foundational knowledge of certain related fields is mandatory. While this book is accessible to all readers, those with some background in the following areas may find it easier to grasp the advanced concepts:

Certification Requirements

To practice and administer Floraopathy™ professionally, it is necessary to become a certified practitioner. Certification ensures you have the knowledge and skills to safely and effectively create and use Floraopathy™ blends for yourself and others. Certification programs typically cover an in-depth understanding of essential oils, safety protocols, blending techniques, and client consultation practices. Completing a recognized certification program will equip you with the expertise needed to practice Floraopathy™ professionally.

Aromatherapy

Understanding the basics of essential oils and their therapeutic uses will provide a solid foundation for learning Floraopathy™. If you are new to aromatherapy, consider taking a beginner's course.

Floraopathy™ – Certificate Course
https://3jinn.com/floraopathy-certificate-course/

Herb/Flower Essence and Homeopathy

Familiarity with herb and flower essences and the principles of homeopathy will enhance your understanding of the vibrational energy healing techniques discussed in this book.

Textbooks and Equipment

While this book aims to be comprehensive on its own, having additional resources and tools can enhance your learning and practice of Floraopathy™. Here are some recommended materials:

Recommended Reading

> *Secrets of a Healer, Magic of Aromatherapy by Dr. Constance Santego*
> *Trade Paperback ISBN: 978-1-7772220-3-1*
> *eBook ISBN 978-1-989013-08-3*

Any books on Aromatherapy: Texts that cover the properties and uses of essential oils.

Any books on Homeopathy and Flower Essences: Resources that provide insight into the principles and applications of these healing modalities.

Equipment for Practical Application

Essential Oils: A variety of high-quality essential oils for creating your own Floraopathy™ blends.

Blending Tools: Dropper bottles, mixing bowls, measuring pipettes, and dark glass storage bottles.

Client Consultation Forms: Standardized forms for documenting personal information and blend formulations, useful for those who wish to practice Floraopathy™ professionally.

Digital Tools

> Access to online resources and communities can provide support and further information as you explore Floraopathy™.

By preparing with these prerequisites and materials, you will be well-equipped to delve into the fascinating world of Floraopathy™ and harness its potential for enhancing your health and well-being. This book will guide you through the process, offering practical tips and insights along the way.

Quick Overview of Aromatherapy

Aromatherapy is the practice of using essential oils extracted from plants to promote physical, emotional, and spiritual well-being. These aromatic compounds have been used in various cultures for their therapeutic properties for thousands of years.

Historical Background

The roots of aromatherapy can be traced back to ancient civilizations such as the Egyptians, Greeks, and Romans. The Egyptians are known to have used essential oils in their embalming practices and religious rituals, while the Greeks and Romans incorporated aromatic oils into their medical treatments, baths, and massages.

In the early 20th century, the term "aromatherapy" was coined by the French chemist René-Maurice Gattefossé, who discovered the healing properties of lavender oil in treating burns. His research and subsequent publications laid the foundation for modern aromatherapy practices.

Principles and Practices

Aromatherapy harnesses the natural essence of plants to address various health concerns. Essential oils are typically extracted through steam distillation or cold pressing and are used in several ways, including:

- Inhalation: Using diffusers, steam inhalations, or inhaler sticks to breathe in the aromatic compounds, which can affect the limbic system in the brain, influencing emotions and memory.

- Topical Application: Diluting essential oils in carrier oils and applying them to the skin for localized treatment or overall therapeutic benefits.
- Bathing: Adding essential oils to bathwater for a relaxing and healing soak.
- Massage: Incorporating essential oils into massage oils to enhance the physical and emotional benefits of the massage.

Therapeutic Benefits

Essential oils are known for their diverse therapeutic properties, which can include:

- Relaxation and Stress Relief: Oils like lavender, chamomile, and bergamot are commonly used to reduce anxiety and promote relaxation.
- Pain Relief: Peppermint, eucalyptus, and ginger oils effectively alleviate headaches, muscle aches, and joint pain.
- Improved Sleep: Lavender and sandalwood oils are often used to promote restful sleep and address insomnia.
- Enhanced Mood and Cognitive Function: Citrus oils like lemon and orange can uplift mood and improve focus and clarity.

Safety Considerations

While aromatherapy offers numerous benefits, it is essential to use essential oils safely. This includes proper dilution, avoiding certain oils during pregnancy, and performing patch tests to check for allergic reactions. Consulting with a qualified aromatherapist or healthcare provider is recommended, especially when using essential oils for therapeutic purposes.

Aromatherapy is a holistic healing practice that leverages the therapeutic properties of essential oils to promote overall well-being. By understanding aromatherapy's history, principles, and benefits, you can incorporate these natural remedies into your daily life to enhance your health and wellness.

How the Science of Aromatherapy Works

Aromatherapy is the practice of using essential oils derived from plants to promote physical, emotional, and spiritual well-being. The science behind aromatherapy involves a complex interaction between the chemical compounds in essential oils and the body's physiological and psychological processes. Here's an overview of how aromatherapy works:

1. Extraction and Composition of Essential Oils

Extraction Methods:

- Steam Distillation: The most common method, where steam is used to extract essential oils from plant material.
- Cold Pressing: Typically used for citrus oils, where the oils are mechanically pressed from the peels.
- Solvent Extraction: Used for delicate flowers, where solvents are used to extract the oils and then the flowers are removed.
- CO_2 Extraction: Carbon dioxide is used under high pressure to extract oils, resulting in a pure, potent product.

Chemical Composition:

- Essential oils are composed of various volatile organic compounds (VOCs) such as terpenes, alcohols, esters, aldehydes, ketones, and phenols. Each oil's unique chemical profile determines its therapeutic properties.

2. Mechanisms of Action

Olfactory System:

- When you inhale essential oils, the scent molecules travel through the nose and stimulate the olfactory receptors. These receptors send signals directly to the olfactory bulb, part of the brain's limbic system.
- The limbic system is involved in emotions, memories, and arousal. This direct pathway explains why scents can evoke strong emotional responses and influence mood and stress levels.

Limbic System:

- The limbic system includes structures such as the amygdala, hippocampus, and hypothalamus, which regulate emotions, memory, and hormone production.
- Inhaling essential oils can stimulate these areas, leading to emotional and physiological effects such as relaxation, mood enhancement, and stress reduction.

Topical Application:

- Essential oils can penetrate the epidermis and enter the bloodstream through dermal absorption when applied to the skin.
- Once in the bloodstream, the chemical compounds can interact with various bodily systems, providing

therapeutic benefits such as anti-inflammatory, analgesic, and antimicrobial effects.

Respiratory System:

- Inhaled essential oils can also impact the respiratory system directly. For example, eucalyptus oil can help open airways and improve breathing by reducing mucus and inflammation in the respiratory tract.

3. Therapeutic Effects

Psychological Effects:

- Stress Reduction: Oils like lavender, bergamot, and chamomile have calming effects, helping to reduce anxiety and stress.
- Mood Enhancement: Citrus oils such as lemon and orange can uplift mood and alleviate symptoms of depression.
- Cognitive Function: Rosemary and peppermint oils can enhance focus, concentration, and memory.

Physiological Effects:

- Anti-inflammatory: Oils like frankincense and ginger can reduce inflammation and pain.
- Antimicrobial: Tea tree and eucalyptus oils have antimicrobial properties that can help fight infections.
- Respiratory Support: Oils such as eucalyptus and peppermint can relieve congestion and improve respiratory function.
- Skin Health: Lavender and tea tree oils can promote wound healing and improve skin conditions like acne and eczema.

Hormonal Effects:

- Some essential oils can influence hormone production and balance. For example, clary sage is known to support hormonal balance in women, especially during menopause.

4. Scientific Research and Evidence

Clinical Studies:

- Numerous studies have demonstrated the efficacy of essential oils in various applications. For instance, lavender oil has been shown to reduce anxiety in preoperative patients, and peppermint oil is effective in treating irritable bowel syndrome (IBS).

In Vitro and In Vivo Studies:

- Laboratory studies on cells and animal models help to elucidate the mechanisms by which essential oils exert their effects, such as their antimicrobial action against bacteria and fungi.

Systematic Reviews and Meta-Analyses:

- Reviews of multiple studies provide a broader understanding of the effectiveness and safety of essential oils. For example, systematic reviews have confirmed the stress-reducing effects of lavender oil.

5. Safety and Precautions

Dilution:

- Essential oils are highly concentrated and should be diluted in a carrier oil before topical application to prevent skin irritation or sensitization.

Allergic Reactions:

- Patch testing is recommended to check for allergic reactions before using a new essential oil.

Quality:

- Use high-quality, pure essential oils from reputable sources to ensure safety and efficacy.

Aromatherapy works through the intricate interaction of essential oil compounds with the body's olfactory, limbic, respiratory, and circulatory systems. The therapeutic effects of essential oils are backed by both traditional use and scientific research, making aromatherapy a powerful tool for promoting overall health and well-being when used safely and appropriately.

Contraindications in Aromatherapy

While Floraopathy™ offers numerous benefits, it's essential to be aware of certain contraindications to ensure the safe and effective use of essential oils. Here are some key considerations for specific populations and health conditions:

Pregnant Women

General Precautions: Pregnant women should be particularly cautious when using essential oils, especially during the first trimester when the risk of miscarriage is higher.

Some essential oils can stimulate uterine contractions or cause other adverse effects.

Oils to Avoid:

- Clary Sage: Can stimulate contractions and should be avoided, especially during the early stages of pregnancy.
- Rosemary: May increase blood pressure and stimulate uterine contractions.
- Sage and Thuja: Can cause bleeding and miscarriage.
- Wintergreen: Contains high levels of methyl salicylate, which can be harmful.
- Basil and Oregano: May be too strong and potentially harmful during pregnancy.
- Safe Oils (with caution):
- Lavender: Generally safe for relaxation and stress relief.
- Chamomile: Can help with relaxation and sleep but should be used in moderation.
- Ylang-Ylang: Useful for stress relief and relaxation but should be used sparingly.

Infants and Young Children

General Precautions: Essential oils should be used with great caution in infants and young children due to their sensitive skin and developing systems.

Always dilute essential oils heavily before use and conduct a patch test.

Oils to Avoid:

- Peppermint: Can cause respiratory issues in young children.
- Eucalyptus: May cause breathing difficulties.

- Wintergreen and Birch: Contain salicylates, which can be harmful.
- Cinnamon and Clove: Highly irritating to the skin and mucous membranes.

Safe Oils (with caution):

- Lavender: Gentle and calming, suitable for use in baths or diluted for topical application.
- Chamomile: Soothing and safe for use in diluted form for skin care and relaxation.
- Tea Tree: Can be used for minor cuts and scrapes but should be highly diluted.

Individuals with Health Conditions

Asthma and Respiratory Issues:

- Essential oils can trigger asthma attacks or exacerbate respiratory issues in some individuals.
- Oils to Avoid: Eucalyptus, rosemary, and peppermint (use with caution).
- Safer Alternatives: Lavender, chamomile, and frankincense (diluted and tested for tolerance).

Epilepsy:

- Certain essential oils can trigger seizures in individuals with epilepsy.
- Oils to Avoid: Rosemary, fennel, sage, and eucalyptus.
- Safer Alternatives: Lavender, chamomile, and ylang-ylang (use with caution and under guidance).

High Blood Pressure:

- Some essential oils can increase blood pressure and should be avoided by individuals with hypertension.
- Oils to Avoid: Rosemary, thyme, and sage.
- Safer Alternatives: Lavender, ylang-ylang, and frankincense (monitor blood pressure and use with caution).

Skin Sensitivities and Allergies:

- Individuals with sensitive skin or allergies should perform a patch test before using any essential oils.
- Common Irritants: Cinnamon, clove, oregano, and lemongrass.
- Gentle Oils: Lavender, chamomile, and tea tree (diluted and tested).

General Guidelines

Consultation: Always consult with a healthcare provider, especially if you have any pre-existing health conditions or are unsure about the safety of a particular essential oil.

Proper Dilution: Essential oils should always be diluted in a carrier oil before topical application to minimize the risk of skin irritation or sensitization.

Patch Testing: Conduct a patch test by applying a small amount of diluted essential oil to the inside of the elbow and waiting 24 hours to check for any adverse reactions.

Quality and Purity: Use high-quality, pure essential oils from reputable sources to ensure safety and effectiveness.

By being mindful of these contraindications and taking appropriate precautions, you can safely incorporate Floraopathy™ into your holistic healing practices and enhance your well-being.

Purpose of a Patch Test

Detailed Guide to Performing a Patch Test for Essential Oils

A patch test is a simple procedure used to determine whether a particular substance, such as an essential oil blend, may cause an allergic reaction or skin sensitivity. This step is crucial because essential oils are highly concentrated and can cause irritation or allergic reactions in some individuals. Performing a patch test ensures that the product is safe for use on your skin, especially when using new or unfamiliar essential oil blends.

Why Perform a Patch Test?

1. Identify Allergic Reactions:
   o Essential oils can cause allergic reactions in some individuals, which may include redness, itching, swelling, or even more severe reactions. A patch test helps identify any potential allergies before applying the product more broadly on your skin.
2. Prevent Skin Irritation:
   o Some essential oils can be irritating to the skin, particularly if you have sensitive skin or if the oil is used in a high concentration. A patch test helps ensure that the blend is diluted appropriately and will not cause irritation.
3. Ensure Safety:
   o Safety is paramount when using essential oils. A patch test is a precautionary measure that

ensures the essential oil blend is safe for your specific skin type.

4. Personal Sensitivity:
    o   Each person's skin can react differently to essential oils. A patch test helps determine your personal sensitivity to the specific blend you are using.

How to Perform a Patch Test

1. Prepare the Test Area:
    o   Choose a small, discrete area of skin to conduct the patch test. Common sites include the inner forearm, behind the ear, or the inside of the elbow. These areas are less likely to be exposed to other substances that could interfere with the test.
2. Clean the Skin:
    o   Ensure the test area is clean and dry. Wash the area with mild soap and water, and then pat it dry with a clean towel.
3. Apply the Essential Oil Blend:
    o   Mix well to ensure the essential oils are properly mixed with the carrier. Apply a small amount (1-2 drops) to the test area.
4. Cover the Area:
    o   You can cover the test area with a bandage or gauze to prevent the oil from rubbing off or being contaminated. This also helps keep the area clean and allows you to monitor it more effectively.
5. Wait and Observe:
    o   Leave the test area uncovered for at least 24 hours. During this period, observe the skin for any signs of redness, itching, swelling, or other adverse reactions.

6. Evaluate the Results:
    o After 24 hours, examine the test area. If there is no reaction, it is generally safe to use the essential oil blend on larger areas of your skin. If you notice any redness, itching, swelling, or other signs of irritation, wash the area immediately with soap and water and discontinue the use of the blend.

What to Do if You Have a Reaction

1. Wash the Area:
    o If you experience any adverse reaction, wash the test area immediately with mild soap and lukewarm water to remove the essential oil.
2. Apply a Soothing Agent:
    o To soothe irritated skin, you can apply a cool compress or an over-the-counter hydrocortisone cream. Aloe vera gel can also help reduce redness and soothe the skin.
3. Avoid Using the Product:
    o Discontinue the use of the essential oil blend and avoid using that particular essential oil in the future.
4. Consult a Healthcare Professional:
    o If the reaction is severe or does not improve, seek medical advice from a healthcare professional.

Performing a patch test is a simple yet crucial step to ensure the safe use of essential oil blend on your skin. By taking this precaution, you can avoid potential allergic reactions or skin irritations, making your aromatherapy experience both safe and enjoyable. Always remember that safety comes first, and a patch test is an effective way to protect your skin and health.

CHAPTER 2: BASICS OF VIBRATIONAL ENERGY HEALING

Subtle Aromatherapy

In many cultures, essential oils are primarily used to address mental or physical problems, often impacting the emotional body. However, there is another lesser-known but important application called subtle aromatherapy. You may or may not encounter subtle aromatherapy or its practitioners, but understanding its principles is valuable.

What is Subtle Aromatherapy?

Subtle aromatherapy utilizes essential oils to influence the subtle body, the psyche, and, as some believe, the soul. This approach focuses on essential oils' energetic or vibrational qualities rather than their physical properties. It operates on the premise that essential oils carry a vibrational frequency that can interact with the body's energy fields to promote healing and balance.

Key Concepts in Subtle Aromatherapy

Subtle Body:

> The subtle body refers to the non-physical aspects of a person, including the aura, chakras, and energy meridians. It is believed that imbalances or blockages in these energy systems can affect physical, emotional, and spiritual health.

Energetic Qualities:

> Essential oils are thought to possess specific vibrational frequencies that resonate with different aspects of the subtle body. By using these oils, practitioners aim to restore balance and harmony to the energy fields.

Psychic and Spiritual Healing:

> Subtle aromatherapy extends beyond physical healing to encompass psychic and spiritual dimensions. It can be used to facilitate personal growth, emotional release, and spiritual connection.

Techniques and Practices in Subtle Aromatherapy

Auric Massage:

> What It Is: Applying essential oils to cleanse and balance the aura, the energy field surrounding the body.

> How to Use: Gently apply diluted essential oils to the body, focusing on sweeping motions that follow the contours of the aura. Oils such as lavender, frankincense, and sage are often used for their purifying properties.

Chakra Balancing:

> What It Is: Using essential oils to harmonize the body's energy centers, known as chakras.

> How to Use: To promote balance and alignment, apply specific essential oils to each chakra point (e.g., rose oil for the heart chakra, sandalwood for the root chakra).

Absent Healing:

> What It Is: Sending healing energy with the aid of essential oils to someone not physically present.

> How to Use: Use visualization and intention, combined with the scent of essential oils, to direct healing energy to a distant person. This can be part of a meditation or prayer practice.

Planetary Healing:

> What It Is: Utilizing essential oils in rituals aimed at healing the Earth.

> How to Use: Perform ceremonies or meditations with essential oils that symbolize love and care for the planet. Oils like cedarwood and patchouli, which are grounding and earthy, can be used in these practices.

Meditation:

> What It Is: Enhancing meditation practices with the supportive energy of essential oils.

> How to Use: Diffuse essential oils or apply them topically before meditation. Oils such as frankincense, sandalwood, and lavender can deepen meditation by promoting relaxation and spiritual connection.

Rituals:

>What It Is: Incorporating essential oils in personal or group rituals for spiritual purposes.

>How to Use: Use essential oils in anointing, blessings, or symbolic actions within rituals. Common oils for rituals include myrrh, frankincense, and rose.

Religious Ceremonies or Services:

>What It Is: Using essential oils in spiritual or religious contexts to deepen the connection to the Divine.

>How to Use: Incorporate essential oils in incense, anointing oils, or sprays used during religious services. Traditional oils such as frankincense and myrrh are often used for their spiritual significance.

Benefits of Subtle Aromatherapy

>Subtle aromatherapy offers a range of benefits that extend beyond physical healing to encompass emotional, spiritual, and energetic well-being. Here's a deeper look at how subtle aromatherapy can support various aspects of health and personal growth:

Emotional Healing

Description: Emotional healing in subtle aromatherapy involves using essential oils to address and release emotional blockages, facilitating emotional balance and resilience.

How It Works: Essential oils interact with the limbic system, the part of the brain responsible for emotions and memories. This interaction can help process and release trapped emotions, reduce stress, and promote a sense of calm and well-being.

Common Oils for Emotional Healing:

- Lavender: Known for its calming and soothing properties, it helps reduce anxiety and stress.
- Rose: Often used for grief and heartache, it promotes feelings of love and compassion.
- Bergamot: Uplifting and energizing, it can help alleviate depression and boost mood.

Applications:

- Inhalation: Diffuse or inhale essential oils directly to quickly influence the emotional state.
- Topical Application: Apply diluted oils to pulse points for sustained emotional support throughout the day.
- Auric Massage: Use essential oils in an auric massage to cleanse and balance the emotional energy field.

Spiritual Growth

Description: Subtle aromatherapy facilitates a deeper connection with the higher self and the Divine, supporting spiritual exploration and growth.

How It Works: The vibrational qualities of essential oils can enhance meditation, prayer, and other spiritual practices, helping to quiet the mind and open the heart to higher states of consciousness.

Common Oils for Spiritual Growth:

- Frankincense: Promotes spiritual awareness and meditation, creating a sacred space for spiritual practices.
- Sandalwood: Calms the mind and encourages deep meditative states.

- Myrrh: Used historically in religious ceremonies, it enhances spiritual connection and grounding.

Applications:

- Meditation: Diffuse essential oils during meditation to deepen the experience and facilitate a connection to the higher self.
- Anointing: Use oils in anointing rituals to symbolize spiritual awakening and dedication.
- Rituals: Incorporate essential oils into spiritual rituals to enhance their significance and effectiveness.

Energetic Balance

Description: Subtle aromatherapy restores harmony to the body's energy fields, promoting overall well-being and vitality.

How It Works: Essential oils resonate with the body's energy centers (chakras) and meridians, helping to clear blockages, balance energies, and enhance the flow of life force (Qi or Prana).

Common Oils for Energetic Balance:

- Geranium: Balances the emotions and harmonizes the energy body.
- Eucalyptus: Clears stagnant energy and enhances respiratory health, which is closely linked to energy flow.
- Juniper: Detoxifies the body and energy field, removing negative energies.

Applications:

- Chakra Balancing: Apply specific essential oils to the chakra points to harmonize the energy centers.

- Energy Healing: Use essential oils in conjunction with practices like Reiki or acupuncture to enhance the flow of energy.
- Aura Cleansing: Perform auric cleansing with essential oils to remove energetic debris and restore clarity.

Support During Transition

Description: Subtle aromatherapy provides comfort and support during times of change and loss, helping individuals navigate transitions with greater ease.

How It Works: Essential oils can stabilize emotions and provide grounding, helping individuals cope with the stress and uncertainty that often accompany major life changes.

Common Oils for Support During Transition:

- Cypress: Assists with letting go and moving forward, making it useful during periods of grief or change.
- Clary Sage: Balances hormones and emotions, supporting women during menstrual cycles, menopause, and other hormonal transitions.
- Patchouli: Grounding and stabilizing, it helps individuals feel secure and centered during times of upheaval.

Applications:

- Inhalation: Use essential oils in a personal inhaler to provide on-the-go support during stressful times.
- Baths: Incorporate essential oils into baths to relax and soothe the body and mind during periods of change.
- Spritzers: Create a spritzer with essential oils to refresh and calm the environment, providing a sense of stability and peace.

Subtle aromatherapy offers profound benefits by addressing the deeper layers of our being—emotional, spiritual, and energetic. The power of subtle aromatherapy lies in the ability of essential oils to touch the mind and spirit in ways that are often beyond verbal expression. Through the careful selection and application of essential oils, practitioners can support their clients in achieving greater balance, growth, and resilience, ultimately enhancing their overall quality of life.

Oils that facilitate a closer connection with the higher self and the Divine, or that provide comfort during times of change and loss, are particularly valued in this practice. By understanding and incorporating subtle aromatherapy, you can enhance your holistic healing practices and promote deeper levels of well-being.

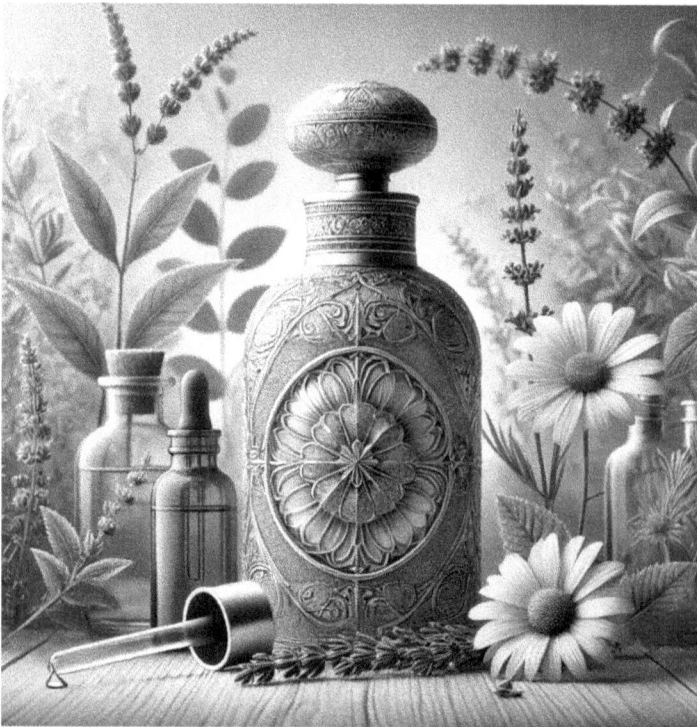

Understanding Herb/Flower Essences/Homeopathy

Introduction to Herb/Flower Essences

Herb and flower essences are natural remedies derived from plants, known for their gentle yet powerful healing properties. These essences capture the vibrational energy of flowers and herbs, which can be used to balance emotional, mental, and spiritual well-being.

What Are Herb/Flower Essences? Herb and flower essences are liquid extracts made from flowers and plants, often preserved in alcohol. Unlike essential oils, which are concentrated aromatic extracts, flower essences are more diluted and work on an energetic level. They are believed to contain the life force or vibrational energy of the plant, which can help to restore balance and harmony within the individual.

How Are They Made? Two primary methods are used to create flower essences:

- o Sun Method: This involves floating flower heads in pure water under direct sunlight for several hours. The water absorbs the vibrational energy of the flowers.
- o Boiling Method: For more robust plants, the flowers are boiled in water to extract their essence. After the energy is transferred to the water, it is mixed with an equal amount of brandy to preserve the essence.

Uses and Benefits Flower essences are used to address a wide range of emotional and spiritual issues. Each flower essence targets specific emotional states or personality traits. For example, Bach's Rescue Remedy, a well-known flower essence blend, is used for stress relief and emotional balance.

Flower essences are typically administered by placing a few drops under the tongue or adding them to water. They can also be used in sprays, baths, or topical applications.

Overview of Homeopathy Principles

Homeopathy is a holistic system of medicine that treats the individual as a whole, rather than focusing solely on specific symptoms. Developed in the late 18th century by German physician Samuel Hahnemann, homeopathy is based on the principle of "like cures like."

Core Principles of Homeopathy

- o Law of Similars: This principle states that a substance that can cause symptoms in a healthy person can also cure similar symptoms in a sick person when administered in highly diluted forms.
- o Potentization: Homeopathic remedies are prepared through a process of serial dilution and succussion (vigorous shaking). This process is believed to enhance the healing properties of the original substance while minimizing side effects.
- o Individualized Treatment: Homeopathy considers the unique physical, emotional, and mental characteristics of the individual. Remedies are selected based on a comprehensive assessment of the patient's overall condition.

Preparation of Remedies Homeopathic remedies are derived from natural substances, including plants, minerals, and animal products. These substances undergo a process of serial dilution, often to the point where no molecules of the original substance remain. Despite this, the energetic imprint of the substance is believed to exert therapeutic effects.

Common Uses and Benefits Homeopathy is used to treat a wide range of conditions, from acute illnesses like colds and flu to chronic conditions such as allergies, arthritis, and mental health issues. Remedies are selected to match the patient's specific symptoms and overall constitution.

Administration and Safety Homeopathic remedies are usually taken orally in the form of small pellets, tablets, or liquid drops. They are generally considered safe and free of significant side effects, making them suitable for individuals of all ages, including pregnant women and infants.

By understanding the principles of herb/flower essences and homeopathy, you can appreciate the foundational elements of vibrational energy healing. Both modalities emphasize the importance of energetic balance and the body's innate ability to heal itself, aligning perfectly with the principles of Floraopathy™.

Edible Carrier Oils and Products in Aromatherapy for Floraopathy™

Edible carrier oils and other products play a significant role in aromatherapy and Floraopathy™. They serve as vehicles for delivering the therapeutic properties of essential oils safely and effectively. Here's an overview of edible carrier oils and other products that can be used in Floraopathy™:

Edible Carrier Oils

1. Olive Oil

- Properties: Olive oil is rich in monounsaturated fats, antioxidants, and vitamins E and K. It has anti-inflammatory and moisturizing properties.
- Uses: It can be used as a carrier oil for internal consumption, skin applications, and massage blends.

2. Coconut Oil

- Properties: Coconut oil contains medium-chain triglycerides (MCTs), which are easily absorbed by the body. It has antibacterial, antifungal, and moisturizing properties.
- Uses: Suitable for both topical and internal use, coconut oil is ideal for cooking, adding to smoothies, and as a carrier oil in massage blends.

3. Sweet Almond Oil

- Properties: Rich in vitamins E and D, as well as fatty acids, sweet almond oil, is known for its soothing and moisturizing effects.
- Uses: It can be used in culinary applications, as a salad dressing, and as a carrier oil for topical applications and massage.

4. Grapeseed Oil

- Properties: Grapeseed oil is high in polyunsaturated fats and antioxidants. It has a light texture and is easily absorbed by the skin.
- Uses: This oil is excellent for salad dressings, cooking, and as a carrier oil in skin care and massage blends.

5. Avocado Oil

- Properties: Avocado oil is rich in oleic acid, potassium, and vitamins A, D, and E. It has anti-inflammatory and healing properties.
- Uses: It is used in cooking, as a dietary supplement, and as a carrier oil for skin care and massage.

6. Sesame Oil

- Properties: Sesame oil contains vitamins E and B complex, as well as minerals like calcium, magnesium, and phosphorus. It has anti-inflammatory and antioxidant properties.
- Uses: Used in culinary applications, as a massage oil, and in skin care products.

7. Sunflower Oil

- Properties: Rich in vitamins A, D, and E, sunflower oil is a light, non-greasy oil that absorbs easily into the skin.
- Uses: It can be used in cooking, as a salad dressing, and as a carrier oil in aromatherapy and skin care blends.

Products in Aromatherapy and Floraopathy™

1. Blends for Internal Use

- Essential Oil Supplements: Some essential oils are safe for internal consumption when diluted properly. For example, peppermint oil can be added to water or taken in a capsule for digestive support.
- Flavored Oils: Edible carrier oils infused with essential oils can be used in culinary applications. For instance, basil-infused olive oil can be used in salads and cooking.

2. Topical Applications

- Massage Oils: Blends of essential oils with edible carrier oils can be used for therapeutic massages. For example, a blend of lavender and sweet almond oil can be used to relax muscles and relieve stress.
- Skin Care Products: Edible carrier oils combined with essential oils can create nourishing skin care products. Coconut oil with tea tree oil can be used as an antibacterial moisturizer.

3. Inhalation Methods

- Diffusers: Essential oils can be diffused into the air for inhalation, providing therapeutic benefits through aromatherapy. Blends of citrus oils with eucalyptus can uplift mood and improve respiratory function.
- Steam Inhalation: Adding a few drops of essential oils like eucalyptus or peppermint to a bowl of hot water for steam inhalation can help clear nasal passages and improve respiratory health.

4. Culinary Uses

- Herbal Teas: Essential oils like peppermint or chamomile can be added to herbal teas for their soothing and digestive properties.
- Cooking: Essential oils like lemon, lime, and basil can enhance the flavor of dishes when used in small quantities.

5. Bath and Body Products

- Bath Oils: Edible carrier oils infused with essential oils can be added to bathwater for a relaxing and therapeutic bath experience.

- Body Butters and Lotions: Combining essential oils with edible carrier oils like coconut oil or shea butter can create luxurious body butters and lotions that nourish the skin.

By understanding the various edible carrier oils and products that can be used in Floraopathy™, you can create versatile and effective blends tailored to your specific needs. These oils and products provide a holistic approach to health and well-being, whether for internal use, topical application, or inhalation.

Other applications for Dosage Guidelines

All dosages are general guidelines, and it's important to remember that more is not necessarily better.

- Bath: Use no more than eight drops of essential oil and less for more potent oils. Use a vegetable solubilizer to help distribute the oil evenly throughout the water.
- Shower: Use two drops or as directed.
- Jacuzzi: Use three drops per person. The essential oil will evaporate quickly due to the hot water, so the primary benefit is through inhalation.
- Wet Sauna: Use two drops per 500-600 ml of water. Limit use to eucalyptus, tea tree, or pine oils, as they are excreted through perspiration.
- Diffusers: Use 1 to 8 drops.
- Kleenex: Use 1 to 2 drops.
- Humidifiers: Use 1 to 9 drops. Be aware that the oil may eventually damage the humidifier.
- Light Rings: Use 4 to 5 drops. Exercise caution due to the fire risk, and it is best to use artificial oils.

All About Hydrosol Water

Hydrosols, also known as floral waters or distillates, are aromatic water solutions obtained from the steam distillation of plants. Unlike essential oils, which are highly concentrated, hydrosols are gentle and contain water-soluble components of the plant, making them suitable for a variety of applications, including some culinary uses.

What is Hydrosol Water?

Production: Hydrosols are produced during the steam distillation process of extracting essential oils. As steam passes through the plant material, it captures both essential oils and water-soluble components. Once the steam condenses back into liquid, the essential oils separate from the water, leaving behind the hydrosol.

Composition: Hydrosols contain micro-drops of essential oils along with the plant's water-soluble compounds. This makes them milder and more suitable for direct skin application and other gentle uses.

Properties: Hydrosols carry the essence of the plant in a diluted form, including its therapeutic properties. They are often used for their soothing, anti-inflammatory, and hydrating effects.

Common Uses of Hydrosols

- Skin Care: Hydrosols are used as toners, facial mists, and ingredients in creams and lotions due to their gentle nature and hydrating properties.
- Aromatherapy: They can be used in diffusers, sprays, and baths for a mild aromatherapeutic effect.

- Household: Hydrosols can be used as natural air fresheners, linen sprays, and gentle cleaners.
- Culinary: Some hydrosols are edible and can be used to flavor foods and beverages.

Edible Hydrosols

While not all hydrosols are suitable for consumption, some are commonly used in culinary applications. Here are a few edible hydrosols:

1. Rose Hydrosol:
   o Flavor: Sweet, floral taste.
   o Uses: Used in desserts, beverages, and as a flavoring in Middle Eastern cuisine. It can also be added to water for a refreshing drink.
2. Orange Blossom (Neroli) Hydrosol:
   o Flavor: Light, citrusy, and floral taste.
   o Uses: Used in pastries, sweets, and beverages. It adds a delicate flavor to culinary dishes and can be used in cocktails and teas.
3. Lavender Hydrosol:
   o Flavor: Floral and slightly sweet.
   o Uses: Can be used in baking, desserts, and beverages. It pairs well with lemon and honey in teas and can be added to lemonade.
4. Peppermint Hydrosol:
   o Flavor: Cool, minty taste.
   o Uses: Used in beverages, desserts, and savory dishes. It is refreshing in drinks and can be added to sauces and salads.
5. Chamomile Hydrosol:
   o Flavor: Mild, apple-like taste.

- Uses: Commonly used in teas, desserts, and as a flavoring for syrups. It has calming properties and is often used in soothing beverages.
6. Lemon Balm (Melissa) Hydrosol:
   - Flavor: Fresh, lemony taste.
   - Uses: Can be added to drinks, desserts, and salads. It has a refreshing flavor and is often used in teas and lemonades.
7. Thyme Hydrosol
   - Flavor: Herbaceous, slightly spicy.
   - Uses: Used in savory dishes, soups, sauces, and marinades. It adds depth and complexity to Mediterranean and French cuisine.
8. Basil Hydrosol
   - Flavor: Fresh, sweet, and slightly peppery.
   - Uses: Can be used in salads, sauces, pestos, and beverages. It pairs well with tomatoes, garlic, and mozzarella.
9. Lemon Verbena Hydrosol
   - Flavor: Bright, lemony, and slightly sweet.
   - Uses: Ideal for flavoring teas, desserts, and cocktails. It adds a refreshing note to fruit salads and sorbets.
10. Coriander Hydrosol
    - Flavor: Citrusy, sweet, and slightly spicy.
    - Uses: Used in Asian and Latin American dishes, soups, and marinades. It complements seafood and chicken dishes well.
11. Ginger Hydrosol
    - Flavor: Warm, spicy, and slightly sweet.
    - Uses: Adds a zing to beverages, desserts, and savory dishes. It is great for ginger teas, stir-fries, and marinades.
12. Spearmint Hydrosol
    - Flavor: Fresh, minty, and slightly sweet.

- o Uses: Perfect for flavoring drinks, desserts, and salads. It can be added to mojitos, iced teas, and fruit salads.
13. Rosemary Hydrosol
    - o Flavor: Herbaceous, pine-like, and slightly bitter.
    - o Uses: Ideal for savory dishes, roasted meats, and vegetables. It pairs well with lamb, potatoes, and bread.
14. Cardamom Hydrosol
    - o Flavor: Warm, sweet, and slightly spicy.
    - o Uses: Used in desserts, beverages, and savory dishes. It adds a unique flavor to chai, rice puddings, and curries.
15. Lemongrass Hydrosol
    - o Flavor: Citrusy, fresh, and slightly herbaceous.
    - o Uses: Popular in Southeast Asian cuisine, it can be used in soups, teas, and marinades. It adds a refreshing flavor to chicken and seafood dishes.
16. Juniper Berry Hydrosol
    - o Flavor: Woody, pine-like, and slightly sweet.
    - o Uses: Can be used in beverages, sauces, and marinades. It is often used in gin and other spirits, as well as in savory dishes.
17. Cucumber Hydrosol
    - o Flavor: Light, fresh, and slightly sweet.
    - o Uses: Ideal for beverages, salads, and cold soups. It adds a refreshing touch to drinks like water, cocktails, and smoothies.
18. Geranium Hydrosol
    - o Flavor: Floral and slightly herbaceous.
    - o Uses: Used in desserts, beverages, and sauces. It pairs well with berries, citrus, and chocolate.

19. Lime Hydrosol
    o Flavor: Bright, citrusy, and slightly tart.
    o Uses: Perfect for beverages, marinades, and desserts. It can be added to water, cocktails, and dressings for a refreshing zing.
20. Bay Laurel Hydrosol
    o Flavor: Herbal, slightly spicy, and woody.
    o Uses: Used in savory dishes, soups, and stews. It adds depth and flavor to Mediterranean and French cuisine.
21. Tarragon Hydrosol
    o Flavor: Anise-like, sweet, and slightly bitter.
    o Uses: Ideal for sauces, dressings, and beverages. It pairs well with chicken, fish, and eggs.
22. Violet Leaf Hydrosol
    o Flavor: Mild, floral, and slightly sweet.
    o Uses: Can be used in desserts, syrups, and beverages. It adds a delicate flavor to sweets and drinks.
23. Clary Sage Hydrosol
    o Flavor: Herbaceous, slightly sweet, and musky.
    o Uses: Used in savory dishes, teas, and desserts. It can enhance the flavor of baked goods and beverages.
24. Anise Hyssop Hydrosol
    o Flavor: Sweet, anise-like, and slightly minty.
    o Uses: Ideal for beverages, desserts, and sauces. It adds a unique flavor to teas, cocktails, and confections.
25. Mugwort Hydrosol
    o Flavor: Herbal, slightly bitter, and aromatic.
    o Uses: Used in traditional dishes, teas, and medicinal recipes. It is often used in Asian cuisine.

26. Cilantro (Coriander) Hydrosol
   o Flavor: Fresh, citrusy, and slightly peppery.
   o Uses: Excellent for adding a bright, fresh flavor to salsas, marinades, and dressings. It can also be used in beverages.
27. Fennel Hydrosol
   o Flavor: Sweet, licorice-like, and slightly earthy.
   o Uses: Can be used in baked goods, soups, and beverages. It adds a unique flavor to teas and confections.
28. Sage Hydrosol
   o Flavor: Earthy, slightly peppery, and aromatic.
   o Uses: Suitable for savory dishes, marinades, and sauces. It pairs well with poultry, pork, and vegetables.
29. Jasmine Hydrosol
   o Flavor: Floral, sweet, and slightly exotic.
   o Uses: Ideal for desserts, teas, and beverages. It can add a luxurious touch to cakes, syrups, and cocktails.
30. Melissa (Lemon Balm) Hydrosol
   o Flavor: Lemon-like, fresh, and slightly sweet.
   o Uses: Great for teas, desserts, and sauces. It can be used to flavor beverages and enhance salads.
31. Bay Leaf Hydrosol
   o Flavor: Herbaceous, slightly spicy, and woody.
   o Uses: Perfect for soups, stews, and sauces. It adds depth to savory dishes, particularly in Mediterranean and French cuisine.
32. Nettle Hydrosol
   o Flavor: Earthy, slightly grassy, and mildly sweet.
   o Uses: Can be used in soups, teas, and smoothies. It adds a nutritious boost to various recipes.

33. Pine Hydrosol
    o Flavor: Fresh, woody, and slightly resinous.
    o Uses: Ideal for beverages, marinades, and desserts. It can be used to create unique cocktails and flavored syrups.
34. Yarrow Hydrosol
    o Flavor: Herbal, slightly bitter, and aromatic.
    o Uses: Suitable for teas, soups, and medicinal recipes. It is often used in traditional herbal preparations.
35. Spikenard Hydrosol
    o Flavor: Earthy, slightly sweet, and musky.
    o Uses: Can be used in teas, desserts, and ceremonial beverages. It adds a unique flavor to drinks and confections.

Hydrosols provide a versatile and gentle way to enjoy the benefits of plants, both in therapeutic and culinary applications. By choosing edible hydrosols, you can add a unique and aromatic touch to your culinary creations while enjoying their subtle health benefits.

How to Make a Hydrosol

Making a hydrosol at home can be a rewarding process. It allows you to create your own aromatic waters from fresh or dried plant material. Here's a step-by-step guide on how to make a hydrosol:

Equipment Needed

- Large pot with a lid (preferably a stainless steel or enamel pot)
- Heat-resistant bowl (to collect the hydrosol)
- Steamer basket or a heat-resistant stand (to keep the plant material above the water)
- Ice (for condensation)
- Fresh or dried plant material
- Water (preferably distilled or purified)
- Clean glass bottles for storage

Step-by-Step Process

1. Prepare the Pot
   - Place the steamer basket or heat-resistant stand at the bottom of the pot.
   - Add enough water to the pot to cover the bottom, but do not touch the steamer basket.
2. Add Plant Material
   - Place the fresh or dried plant material on the steamer basket or stand. Make sure the plant material is not submerged in water.
   - Common plants used for hydrosols include lavender, rose, chamomile, peppermint, and rosemary.

3. Place the Bowl
   o Put the heat-resistant bowl on top of the plant material. This bowl will collect the hydrosol as it drips down from the lid.
4. Invert the Lid
   o Place the lid on the pot upside down. This will allow the steam to condense on the lid and drip into the bowl.
   o You can place ice on top of the inverted lid for better condensation. The ice helps cool the steam, turning it back into liquid.
5. Heat the Pot
   o Turn on the stove and heat the pot. Allow the water to simmer gently. Avoid boiling, as high heat can destroy the delicate aromatic compounds.
   o Keep an eye on the ice and replace it as it melts to maintain the cooling effect.
6. Collect the Hydrosol
   o As the steam rises, it will pass through the plant material, capturing the aromatic compounds.
   o The steam will condense on the cold lid and drip into the bowl, forming the hydrosol.
7. Cool and Store
   o Once you have collected enough hydrosol (this can take 30 minutes to 2 hours), turn off the heat and allow the pot to cool.
   o Carefully remove the bowl with the hydrosol.

Transfer the hydrosol to clean glass bottles using a funnel. Label the bottles with the date and type of hydrosol.

Store the hydrosol in a cool, dark place, preferably in the refrigerator, to maintain its freshness and extend its shelf life.

Tips for Making Hydrosols

- Use Fresh Plant Material: Whenever possible, use fresh plant material for a more potent hydrosol. If using dried material, ensure it is of high quality.
- Sterilize Equipment: Sterilize all equipment before use to prevent contamination.
- Keep an Eye on Water Level: Ensure the water level in the pot does not drop too low. Add more water if necessary to prevent burning the pot or plant material.
- Small Batches: Make small batches of hydrosol to ensure it remains fresh and effective.

By following these steps, you can create your own high-quality hydrosols at home, capturing the essence of your favorite plants in a versatile and aromatic form.

CHAPTER 3: BASICS OF THERAPEUTIC CROSS REFERENCING

The following are taught in detail in Dr. Santego's "Floraopathy™ Certificate Course" through 3Jinn Business Hub.

The basics of how to use Therapeutic Cross-Referencing for the Floraopathy Blends:

Therapeutic cross-referencing is a powerful technique used in Floraopathy™ to create highly effective and personalized essential oil blends. This method involves combining various therapeutic properties of essential oils to address multiple conditions or symptoms simultaneously. Here's an overview of the basics of cross-referencing for blends:

1. Identify the Main Condition or Symptom:
    a. Start by determining the primary condition or symptom that needs addressing. This could be anything from physical ailments like headaches or muscle pain to emotional issues like anxiety or stress.
2. Select Secondary Conditions or Symptoms:
    a. Choose up to two additional conditions or symptoms that may be related to or contributing to the main issue. For example, if the primary condition is stress, secondary

conditions might include insomnia and digestive discomfort.

3. Choose Appropriate Essential Oils:
   a. For each condition or symptom, select essential oils known for their therapeutic benefits. Each oil should be chosen based on its properties and how it can contribute to alleviating the specific conditions identified.
   b. Consider oils that offer multiple benefits. For instance, lavender is known for its calming effects, pain relief, and ability to improve sleep quality.

4. Organize Oils into Blends:
   a. Organize the selected essential oils into blends that can address all identified conditions. Ensure that each blend is balanced, with top, middle, and base notes if you are creating an aromatic blend. This helps in creating a well-rounded and effective mixture.
   b. For example, a blend for stress relief might include lavender (top note), chamomile (middle note), and frankincense (base note).

5. Check for Contraindications:
   a. Before finalizing any blend, cross-check the essential oils for any contraindications. Some oils may not be suitable for certain individuals, especially those with allergies, pregnant women, or those with specific health conditions.
   b. Ensure the safety of the blend by verifying that all chosen oils are compatible with each other and safe for the intended use.

6. Formulate the Blend:
   a. Once you have selected and organized your oils, formulate the blend by combining the essential oils in appropriate proportions. Start with a

        small batch to test the effectiveness and adjust as needed.

    b. Use precise measurements to maintain consistency in the blend's therapeutic effects.

7. Application Methods:

    a. Determine the best method of application for the blend. This could be through diffusion, topical application, or creating a spritzer or bath blend. The method of application can enhance the effectiveness of the blend.

For instance, a blend for respiratory issues might be best used in a diffuser, while a blend for muscle pain could be applied topically.

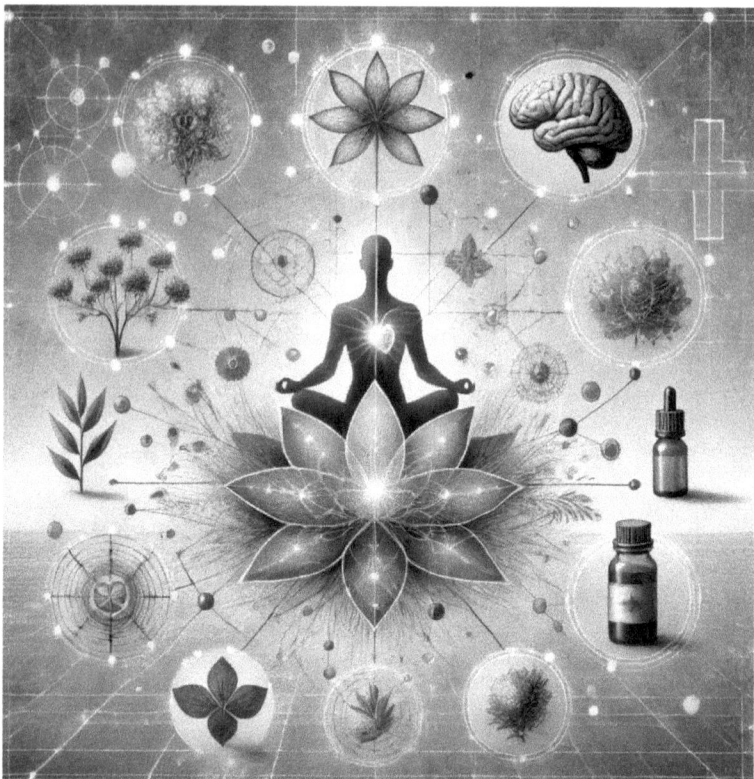

For a more comprehensive guide on creating and using therapeutic cross-referenced blends, refer to Dr. Constance Santego's book **"Secrets of a Healer – Magic of Aromatherapy."** This book provides detailed instructions, advanced techniques, and numerous examples to help you master the art of blending essential oils for holistic healing.

Trade Paperback ISBN: 978-1-7772220-3-1
eBook ISBN 978-1-989013-08-3

Certificate Course Information:
https://3jinn.com/floraopathy-certificate-course/

CHAPTER 4: CREATING FLORAOPATHY™ BLENDS

Creating Floraopathy™ blends is an art that combines knowledge of essential oils, an understanding of vibrational energy, and intuitive skills to create personalized and effective remedies. This module will guide you through the essential steps and considerations in creating these unique blends.

1st Step: Client Consultation and Form Completion

Understanding Client Needs

The first step in creating a Floraopathy™ blend is to thoroughly understand the client's needs. This involves a detailed consultation to gather information about the client's physical, emotional, and spiritual state. Here are the key elements to consider:

1. Physical Health: Discuss any physical ailments or conditions the client is experiencing. This includes chronic illnesses, acute symptoms, and overall physical well-being.
2. Emotional State: Explore the client's emotional health, including stress levels, anxiety, depression, and any other emotional challenges.
3. Spiritual Well-being: Consider the client's spiritual needs and goals. This might involve discussing their spiritual practices, beliefs, and any spiritual challenges they are facing.

Completing the Client Form

A well-structured client form is essential for documenting the information gathered during the consultation. The form should include sections for:

- Personal information (name, age, contact details)
- Health history and current physical conditions
- Emotional health assessment
- Spiritual health assessment
- Specific goals for the Floraopathy™ treatment

By thoroughly completing the client form, you ensure that all relevant information is considered when creating the blend.

2nd Step: Formulating a Blend

Selecting Essential Oils

The next step is to select the essential oils that will be used in the blend. This selection should be based on the information gathered during the consultation and the therapeutic properties of the oils. Here are some key considerations:

1. Therapeutic Properties: Choose oils that have properties that match the client's needs. For example, lavender is known for its calming effects, while peppermint is invigorating and can help with headaches.
2. Synergy: Consider how the oils work together. Some oils have synergistic effects when combined, enhancing their overall therapeutic benefits.
3. Safety: Ensure the selected oils are safe for the client, considering any allergies, sensitivities, or contraindications.

Creating the Blend

Once the oils are selected, it's time to create the blend. Here are the steps involved:

1. Determine Proportions: Decide on the proportions of each oil in the blend. A common ratio is to use three to five different oils, with one or two dominant oils and the others in supporting roles.
2. Mixing: Combine the oils in a clean, dark glass bottle. Dark glass helps protect the oils from light, preserving their potency.
3. Dilution: If the blend is intended for topical use, dilute it with a carrier oil such as jojoba, almond, or coconut oil. A typical dilution ratio is 2-5% essential oil to carrier oil.

Testing the Blend

Before using the blend, it's important to test it for effectiveness and any adverse reactions. Apply a small amount to the client's skin and observe for any irritation or allergic reactions. Additionally, evaluate the blend's therapeutic effects and adjust if necessary.

Storage and Use

Store the blend in a cool, dark place to maintain its potency. Provide the client with instructions on how to use the blend, including application methods and frequency of use.

Creating Floraopathy™ blends is a deeply personal and intuitive process that requires understanding both the science of essential oils and the unique needs of each client.

CHAPTER 5: FLORAOPATHY PROCEDURE

Creating Detailed Floraopathy™ Blends

As in the Aromatherapy Standard course, creating Floraopathy™ blends involves a structured process to ensure the selection of the most appropriate essential oils for addressing specific needs. This process includes the use of a form to systematically choose your Essential Oils (ESO) and refine the blend. Here's a more detailed guide on how to create Floraopathy™ blends:

Step-by-Step Guide to Creating Floraopathy™ Blends

STEP 1: BLENDING FORM

Use a Form to Choose Your Essential Oils (ESO)

The first step is to use a Therapeutic Cross Referencing form to document the selection process for your essential oils. This form helps ensure a comprehensive approach to creating a personalized blend.

1. **Stress is the Main Condition**
   o Stress is always the main condition!
2. **Choose Two More Conditions**
   Physical/Emotional/Mental/Spiritual
   o Select two additional conditions. These can be from any of the following categories:
      ▪ **Physical:** Conditions affecting the body, such as pain, inflammation, or fatigue.
      ▪ **Emotional:** Additional emotional states, such as fear, happiness, or frustration.
      ▪ **Mental:** Conditions related to the mind, such as concentration, clarity, or confusion.
      ▪ **Spiritual:** Aspects affecting the spirit, such as spiritual grounding, connection, or growth.
3. Write in the appropriate Top, Middle, and Base (TMB) Essential Oils Under Each Condition.
   • List the potential essential oils known for their therapeutic benefits in each chosen condition.
4. **Check and Cross Out Any Contra-Indications**
   • Review the list of potential essential oils and _**cross out**_ any contraindications for the client. This might include allergies, sensitivities, or specific health conditions that make certain oils unsuitable.

In the Floraopathy Course, all of this is taught in detail.

Configure the client's *Therapeutic Cross Referencing (TCR)* blend.

Main Condition			Secondary Condition			Third Condition		
Stress								
Top	Mid	Base	Top	Mid	Base	Top	Mid	Base
Bas	Cha	Ben						
Ber	Ger	C/W						
C/S	Hys	Fra						
Lem	Jun	Imm						
Man	Lav	Jas						
Ora	Mar	L/B						
Pet	Pep	Myr						
Thy	Pin	Ner						
Yar	R/M	Pat						
	R/W	Ros						
		S/W						
		Vet						
		Y/Y						

Contra-Indications:							
Hydrosol Water:							
Stabilizer: Alcohol (type) Vodka____ Brandy____ , Vegetable____ or Witch Hazel							
Oil	Oil	Oil	Oil		Oil	Oil	Oil
# of Drops	# of Drops	# of Drops ____	# of Drops ____		# of Drops ____	# of Drops	# of Drops ____

STEP 2: MASTER BLEND

Floraopathy™ Master Blend

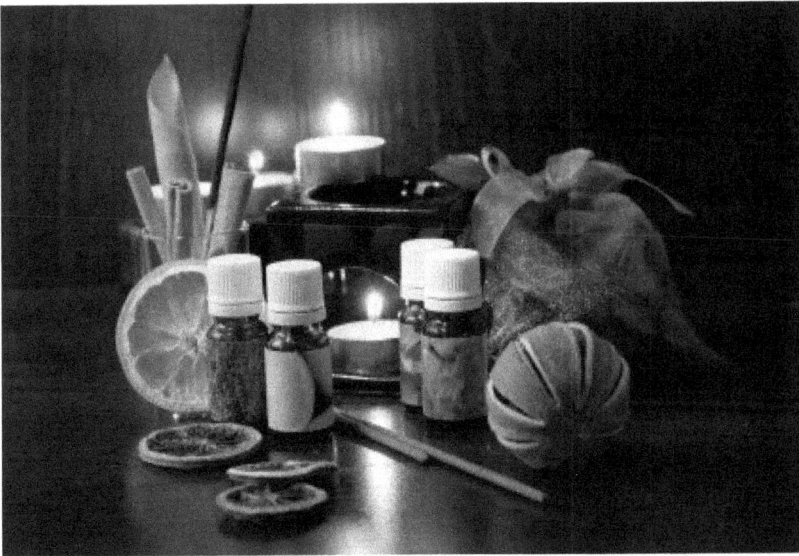

Create the Floraopathy™ Master Blend

Choose Your Essential Oils to Use

1. From the TCR answers, Muscle Testing for the best choice of Essential Oils
   - Muscle Testing Basics: Muscle testing, also known as applied kinesiology, is a technique used to determine the body's response to various substances. It can help identify which essential oils are most beneficial for the client.
   - Testing Process: Test one essential oil at a time. Have the client hold the oil bottle or a diluted sample while they perform a simple muscle test. This might involve the client holding their arm

out and resisting gentle pressure applied by the practitioner. A strong response indicates a positive reaction, while a weak response indicates the opposite.

- o Select Up to Seven Oils: Continue muscle testing until you have identified one to a maximum of seven essential oils that elicit a strong, positive response.

By following this detailed process, you can create highly personalized and effective Floraopathy™ blends. The use of muscle testing ensures that each blend is specifically tailored to the client's unique energetic needs, providing optimal therapeutic benefits. This method combines scientific knowledge with intuitive practice, making Floraopathy™ a powerful tool for holistic healing.

Rules To Creating The Blend

The Master Blend's total number of drops should never exceed *"twelve"* drops!

- Four drops of a Top Note essential oil equals four (4) drops.
- Three drops of a Middle Note equals four (4) drops of a Top Note.
- One (1) drop of a Base Note is equal to the four (4) drops of a Top Note or three (3) drops of a Middle Note.

Blending Formulas/Recipes:

Diseases, illnesses, or conditions are often classified as either chronic or acute.

- Chronic: A chronic disease, illness, or condition that is long-lasting or recurring. It tends to develop slowly and persist over time. An example of a chronic condition is Chronic Fatigue Syndrome.
- Acute: An acute disease, illness, or condition develops rapidly and typically resolves quickly. An example of an acute condition is a common cold, which often appears suddenly and resolves within about 14 days.

Blending essential oils for these conditions can be categorized into three types of formulas:

I. Chronic Blends:
   - Use this formula for long-lasting or recurring conditions:
   - Formula: Middle (3 drops), Middle (3 drops), Base (1 drop) = 7 drops.
II. Acute Blends:
   - Use this formula for conditions that develop and resolve quickly:
   - Formula: Top (4 drops), Middle (3 drops), Middle (3 drops) = 10 drops.
III. Synergistic Blends:
   - This blend is ideal for addressing a wide range of conditions. "Synergistic" means that the combined effect of the oils is greater than the sum of their individual effects. The oils work together to enhance each other's properties, creating a more effective blend.

    o Formula: Top (4 drops), Middle (3 drops), Base (1 drop) = 8 drops.

These formulas ensure that the essential oils are blended to maximize their therapeutic benefits for both chronic and acute conditions.

Top notes are absorbed by the body quickly but also evaporate rapidly. In contrast, base notes take longer to be absorbed but have a much longer-lasting effect.

BLENDING MEASUREMENTS

Measurement Guide for Essential Oil Blends

When discussing blends and measuring our oils, we generally use milliliters. Here is a handy conversion guide:

1. 1 teaspoon = 5 ml (0.2 oz)
2. 1 dessertspoon = 10 ml (0.34 oz)
3. 1 tablespoon = 15 ml (0.5 oz)
4. 30 ml = 1 oz

Bottles and other containers should have their size marked on the bottom. The following measurement conversion chart is for your information and will vary depending on the oil thickness.

Drops	tsp.	oz.	dram		ml.
10	1/10	1/60	about 1/8		about ½
12.5	1/8	1/48	1/6		about 5/8
25	¼	1/24	1/3		about 1 ¼
50	½		1/12	2/3	about 2 ½
100	1	1/6	1 1/3		about 5
150	1 ½	¼	2		about 13.5
300	3	½	4		about 15
600	6	1	8		about 30
24	8	4	1/2		
48	16	8	1		1/2
96	32	16	2		1

Three Recipe Choices for the Master Blend

SYNERGISTIC RECIPE

If possible, this blend is best. It acts fast (Top) and lasts a long time (Middle and Base).

Synergistic Blend: Four drops of a top note, three drops of a middle note, and one drop of a base note are the maximum for this blend *(drops used equals eight (8))*.

> **Blend recipe for one (1) use**
> **T M B**
> **4 3 1 (drops)**
>
> *Blend recipe for ten (10) uses*
>
> **5 ml bottle (holds 100 drops)**
>
> *Top: 50 drops = 2 ml + 10 dr*
>
> *Middle: 37.5 drops = 1 ml + 17 1/2dr*
>
> *Base: 17.5 drops*

Important Note: It is generally not recommended, but if you must use more than one base note, limit it to a maximum of three drops per blend. No additional drops can be added beyond this limit.

ACUTE RECIPE (for a condition under one year)

Blend recipe for one (1) use.
T M M
4 3 3 (drops)

Blend recipe for ten (10) uses

A 5 ml bottle (holds 100 drops)

Top: 40 drops = 2 ml

Middle: 30 drops = 1.5 ml

Middle: 30 drops = 1.5 ml

CHRONIC RECIPE (for a condition over one year)

Blend recipe for one (1) use.
M M B
3 3 1 (drops)

Blend recipe for ten(10) uses

5 ml bottle (holds 100 drops)

Middle: 43 drops = 2 ml + 3 dr

Middle: 43 drops = 2 ml + 3 dr

Base: 14 drops = .5 ml + 4 dr

Comparing the Potency of Essential Oils to Alcohol

Imagine the potency of essential oils in a way that's similar to alcohol. You don't need as much to achieve the same effect.

- o Beer, about 5% alcohol (Comparable to a Top Note).
- o Wine, with about 12% alcohol (Comparable to Middle Notes).
- o Spirits like gin, vodka, rum, or tequila, with about 40% alcohol (Comparable to Base Note).

Just as you would need to drink a lot more beer than spirits to reach the same level of alcohol, you need far less of a base note to achieve a significant effect.

Step 2: Master Blend Recipe

Use only steam-distilled essential oils (ESO). *Note: Absolute essential oils are too concentrated for this process.*

1. Mix the (Synergistic, Acute, or Chronic) blend from the TCR form in a glass beaker.

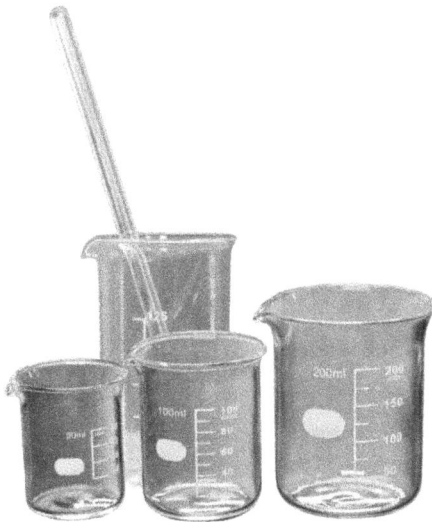

2. Stir the blend thoroughly.
3. Transfer **_one drop_** of the Master Blend to "another" glass container.

4. Use the "remaining mixture" to create a "carrier-based" product, such as:
    - A Massage Oil Aromatherapy Blend
    - A Cream Based Aromatherapy Blend

Body Cream

- 25 ml Cream (unscented is best)
- Add the remaining Master Blend and stir
- Labeling the contents of the container is legally required

OR...

Massage Oil

- Carrier oil (your choice – grapeseed, olive, etc.) 25 ml – 60 ml for one body massage
- Add the remaining Master Blend and stir
- Labeling the contents of the container is legally required

See the full recipes under "RECIPES."

Usage Guidelines for Essential Oil Blends

The maximum essential oil blend for one-time use in a day is the recipe for an acute, chronic, or synergistic blend. For every 25 mL (*or more*) of carrier oil, cream, or spritzer, you can add the specified amount of top (T), middle (M), or base (B) note drops.

STEP 3: INITIAL DILUTION

Floraopathy™ Bath Blend

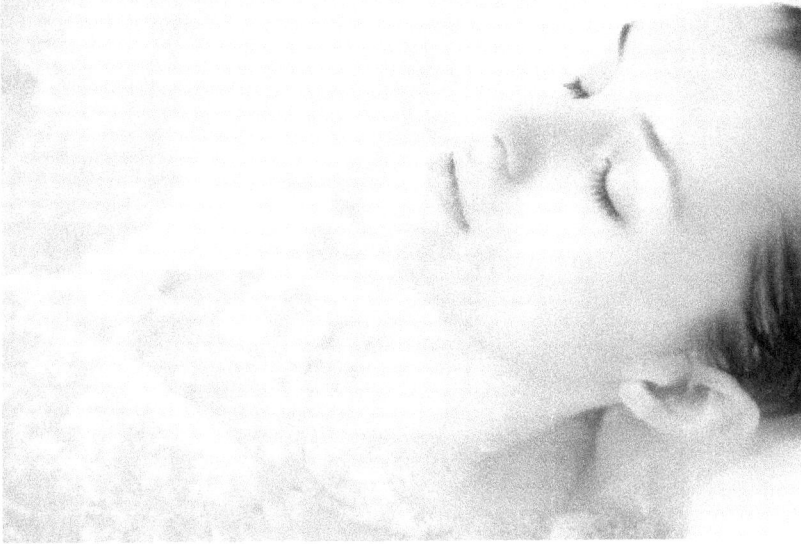

Initial Dilution in a New Glass Container

1. Add a single drop of the **"Master Blend"** *(original blend)*.
2. Add ½ teaspoon of stabilizer (vodka, brandy, vegetable, or witch hazel).
3. Add 60 ml of distilled water.
4. Stir well for 1-5 minutes or shake well in a sealed container.
5. Transfer ***one drop*** of this **Initial Dilution** to a "third" glass container.

Use the remaining mixture to create a carrier-based product, such as:

- An Aromatherapy Bath Blend

STEP 4: SECONDARY DILUTION

Floraopathy™ Spritzer Blend

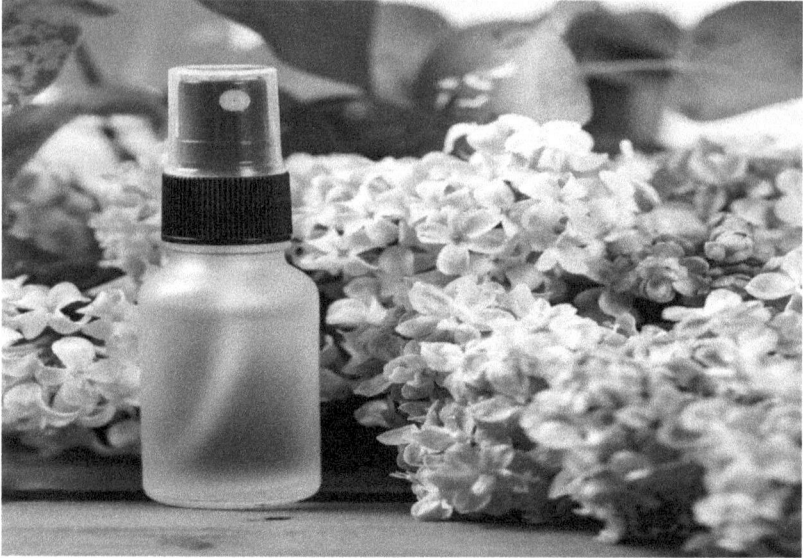

Secondary Dilution in a New Glass Container

1. Shake the previous blend well.
2. Add one (1) drop from the "Initial Dilution."
3. Add ½ tsp of stabilizer.
4. Add 120 mls distilled water.
5. Stir well for 1-5 minutes or shake well in a sealed container.
6. Transfer ***one drop*** of this **Secondary Dilution** to a "fourth" glass container that has an eye dropper.

Use the remainder of the mixture to make a spritzer for:

- A Subtle or Spiritual Application.

Note: When using the spritzer, shake well. ***Remove your glasses***, spray in front of you, and walk into the mist.

STEP 5: FLORAOPATHY™ ORAL BLEND

Floraopathy™ Oral Blend

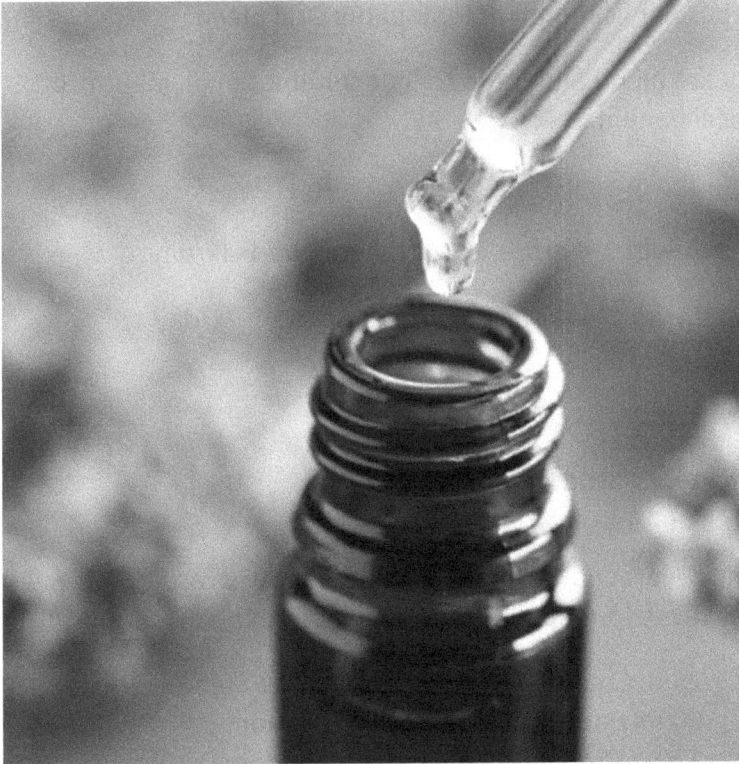

Third and last Dilution in a New Glass Container

1. Shake the previous blend well.
2. Combine all in a glass bottle with an "eye dropper" lid.
3. Add one (1) drop from the "**Secondary Dilution.**"
4. Add 60 mls of distilled water.

The final diluted blend is now ready for use.

Dosages:

Floraopathy™ Oral Blend

Dropper Application for Floraopathy Oral Blend:

Apply the blend under the tongue for emotional, mental, or physical benefits.

> Shake well!
>
> Adult: 1-4 drops under the tongue 1-4x/day
>
> Child: 1-4 drops under the tongue 1-2x/day

Session Outline

During a Floraopathy™ session, the client will receive and follow these four applications to complete their treatment:

1. 25ml Cream/Oil Blend from Master Blend
2. 60 ml Bath Blend from Initial Dilution
3. 120 ml Spritzer Blend from Secondary Dilution
4. 60 ml Floraopathy™ Oral Blend

Session Overview:

1. Initial Consultation:
   - The client arrives, and you gather comprehensive health information.
2. Based on this information, you prepare a custom blend (Synergistic, Acute, or Chronic) before the client's next visit.
3. Follow-Up Session:
   - The client can receive a treatment session (massage, reflexology, etc.) using their personalized Master Blend during the next session.
   - Or they can just pick up their blends for home use.
4. Home Application:
   - The client will take home the remaining applications to complete over a specified period:
     - **Cream/Oil Blend:** to be rubbed on the body *(if not used in the follow-up session)*.
     - **Bath:** Take one therapeutic bath using the blend within seven (7) days.
     - **Spritzer:** Use the spritzer 1-5 times daily for seven (7) days.
     - **Dropper Application:** Administer the dropper application under the tongue for two weeks.

This structured approach ensures a comprehensive and personalized treatment plan, leveraging the benefits of Floraopathy™ both in session and at home.

Labeling the Bottles

FLORAOPATHY™ MASTER BLEND
Client Blend ESO

———— ———— ————
        ____mls
Use cream or oil blend as needed
www.floraopathy.com

FLORAOPATHY™ BATH BLEND
Client Bath Blend

———— ———— ————
        120mls
Pour full content into a tub
Of warm water
www.floraopathy.com

FLORAOPATHY™ SPRITZER BLEND
S Blend Client Spritzer

———— ———— ————
        60 mls
Remove glasses, spray in front
of you, and walk into the mist
as needed
www.floraopathy.com

FLORAOPATHY™ ORAL BLEND
E M S P Client Blend

———— ———— ————
        60mls
Dose: Apply under the tongue
Adult: 1-4 drops 1-4x/day
Child: 1-4 drops 1-2x/day
www.floraopathy.com

CHAPTER 6: HOW TO MUSCLE TEST

Muscle testing, also known as applied kinesiology, is a technique used to evaluate the body's response to various substances, including essential oils, by assessing muscle strength. This method helps determine which essential oils are most beneficial for the client and the optimal amount to use in a Floraopathy™ blend.

The Basics of Muscle Testing

1. Preparation
   o Ensure the client is relaxed and hydrated. Muscle testing works best when the body is in a balanced state.
   o The client should be seated or standing in a comfortable position.
2. Choosing a Test Muscle
   o Select a muscle to test, commonly the deltoid muscle in the upper arm. This muscle is easy to access and provides reliable results.
   o Have the client extend their arm to the side, parallel to the ground.
3. Baseline Test
   o Establish a baseline by gently pressing down on the client's extended arm while they resist the pressure. This initial test helps you understand the client's natural muscle strength.

- o Ensure the client can resist your pressure without too much difficulty, indicating a strong muscle response.
4. Testing Essential Oils
    - o Have the client hold the bottle of essential oil or a diluted sample in their opposite hand, close to their body.
    - o Repeat the muscle test by applying the same amount of pressure to the client's extended arm while they resist.
5. Interpreting Results
    - o A strong response (the client can resist the pressure) indicates a positive reaction to the essential oil, suggesting it is beneficial for the client.
    - o A weak response (the client cannot resist the pressure) indicates a negative reaction, suggesting the oil may not be suitable.

Example of Muscle Testing Process

1. Baseline Test:
    - o The client extends their arm.
    - o The practitioner presses down, and the client resists.
    - o Establish the natural muscle strength.
2. Testing Essential Oils:
    - o The client holds Lavender oil.
    - o The practitioner presses down on the extended arm while the client resists.
    - o If the arm remains strong, lavender is beneficial.
    - o Repeat this for other oils like lemon and basil.
3. Testing for Drop Count:
    - o The client holds Lavender oil.
    - o The practitioner tests with the client, thinking of 1 drop, 2 drops, etc.

o If the arm remains strong at 5 drops, that is the optimal amount.

Reference for Further Learning

For a more comprehensive understanding of muscle testing, including advanced techniques and applications, refer to Dr. Constance Santego's book, **"Secrets of a Healer – Magic of Muscle Testing."** This book provides detailed instructions, case studies, and practical tips to master the art of muscle testing, enhancing your practice of Floraopathy™ and other holistic healing methods.

By incorporating muscle testing into your practice, you can create highly personalized and effective Floraopathy™ blends that align with the client's unique energetic needs, ensuring optimal therapeutic benefits.

CHAPTER 7: RECIPES

Creating a Floraopathy™ Cream Blend

Ingredients:

- 25mls or more of unscented cream base (e.g., shea butter, aloe vera gel, or a natural moisturizer)
- Essential oils from New Directions Aromatics (selected based on Therapeutic Cross Referencing, TCR)
- Optional: Vitamin E oil (for added skin benefits and preservation)

Equipment:

- Mixing bowl
- Measuring spoons
- Whisk or spoon
- Clean, sterilized jar for storage

Instructions:

1. **Select Your Essential Oils**:
   - Use TCR to choose essential oils based on the desired therapeutic effects.
2. **Mix Essential Oils with Cream Base**:
   - In a mixing bowl, add the selected essential oils to the unscented cream base.
   - Stir thoroughly to ensure the oils are well incorporated into the cream.

3. **Add Optional Vitamin E Oil**:
   - o Add a few drops of vitamin E oil to the mixture for its skin benefits and preservative qualities.
   - o Mix well.
4. **Store the Cream**:
   - o Transfer the mixture to a clean, sterilized jar with a tight-fitting lid.
   - o Label the jar with the date, ingredients used, and number of drops.
5. **Use the Cream**:
   - o Apply the cream to your skin as needed, avoiding sensitive areas like the eyes.
   - o Store in a cool, dark place to preserve the integrity of the essential oils.

Creating a Floraopathy™ Oil Blend

Ingredients:

- 25 mls or more of a carrier oil (e.g., jojoba oil, sweet almond oil, or coconut oil)
- Essential oils from New Directions Aromatics (selected based on Therapeutic Cross Referencing, TCR)
- Optional: Vitamin E oil (for added skin benefits and preservation)

Equipment:

- Small glass bottle with a dropper or pump top
- Measuring spoons
- Funnel (optional, for easier pouring)

Instructions:

1. **Select Your Essential Oils**:
   - Use TCR to choose essential oils based on the desired therapeutic effects.
2. **Prepare the Carrier Oil**:
   - Measure 25 mls or more of your chosen carrier oil and pour it into a small glass bottle.
3. **Add Essential Oils to the Carrier Oil**:
   - Using a dropper, add the essential oils to the carrier oil.
   - **Note**: For a 2% dilution (safe for most adults), use approximately (12) drops of essential oil per ounce of carrier oil. Adjust the number of drops based on your blend's strength and intended use.
4. **Add Optional Vitamin E Oil**:
   - Add a few drops of vitamin E oil for its skin benefits and preservative qualities.
   - Mix well.
5. **Mix and Store**:
   - Cap the bottle tightly and shake gently to mix the oils.
   - Label the bottle with the date and ingredients used.
   - Store in a cool, dark place to preserve the integrity of the essential oils.
6. **Use the Oil Blend**:
   - Apply a small amount of the oil blend to the skin, massaging gently. Avoid using near sensitive areas like the eyes.
   - Use as needed for massage, moisturizing, or targeted application.

Tips for Creating Floraopathy™ Cream and Oil Blends

- **Quality Ingredients**: Use high-quality, pure essential oils and carrier oils from reputable sources like New Directions Aromatics to ensure the best therapeutic benefits.
- **Patch Test**: Perform a patch test before using a new blend to check for skin sensitivity or allergic reactions.
- **Proper Dilution**: Follow recommended dilution guidelines to ensure safety and efficacy, especially for sensitive skin areas or children.
- **Clean Tools**: Use clean, sterilized tools and containers to prevent contamination and preserve the blend's quality.

By following these steps, you can create personalized Floraopathy™ cream and oil blends that cater to your specific needs and preferences, enhancing your skincare and therapeutic routines.

Creating a Floraopathy™ Bath Blend

Creating a bath blend with essential oils can enhance your bathing experience, providing therapeutic benefits and relaxation. Here's a step-by-step guide to making your own bath blend:

Ingredients

- One (1) drop from the Master Blend
- 60 mls of water
- Vegetable Solubilizer (optional): Helps distribute essential oils evenly in the water.
- 1 -2 cups of Epsom Salts or Sea Salt (optional): for additional therapeutic benefits and to help disperse the oils in the water.

Equipment

- Small mixing bowl
- Measuring spoons
- Whisk or spoon
- Glass jar or bottle for storage

Step-by-Step Instructions

1. In a small glass container, combine one drop of the Master Blend with 60mls of water.
2. Stir gently to blend the oils.
3. Optional: Add a Vegetable Solubilizer
   - You can add a vegetable solubilizer to your blend to ensure the essential oils disperse evenly in the water. *Follow the manufacturer's instructions for the appropriate ratio.*
   - Mix well to combine.
4. Optional: Add Epsom Salts or Sea Salt

5. Store Your Bath Blend
   - Transfer the bath blend to a glass jar or bottle with a tight-fitting lid.
   - Label the container with the date and the ingredients used.
6. Use Your Bath Blend
   - When ready to use, add the bath blend to your running bathwater.
   - If using salts, pour them directly under the running water to help dissolve them.
   - Stir the water with your hand to ensure the oils are evenly dispersed.
   - Soak in the bath for at least 20-30 minutes to fully enjoy the therapeutic benefits.

Tips for a Therapeutic Bath

- **Test for Skin Sensitivity**: Before using the bath blend, do a patch test to ensure you don't have any adverse reactions to the essential oils.
- **Hydrate**: Drink water before and after your bath to stay hydrated.
- **Relaxation**: Create a calming environment by dimming the lights, playing soft music, or lighting candles.

By following these steps, you can create a personalized bath blend that enhances your bath experience and provides targeted therapeutic benefits.

Creating a Floraopathy™ Spritzer Blend

Creating a Floraopathy™ spritzer is an easy and effective way to enjoy the benefits of essential oils throughout your day. Spritzers can be used for various purposes, such as refreshing your space, calming your mind, or invigorating your senses.

Ingredients

1. 120 mls of distilled water (or hydrosol if preferred)
2. Witch hazel (optional, helps emulsify the oils and water)
3. Vegetable glycerin (optional, adds a moisturizing effect)
4. Glass spray bottle (4 oz)

Equipment

- Measuring spoons or pipette
- Small funnel (optional, for easier pouring)
- Stirring stick or small whisk

Instructions

1. Prepare the Spray Bottle
   - Pour just enough to cover the bottom of a container with either; witch hazel, vegetable solubilizer, or alcohol.
2. Using a small funnel, pour the distilled water (or hydrosol) into the glass spray bottle, filling it half way.
3. Add one (1) drop from the Initial Dilution (Bath Blend)
4. Fill the bottle to almost full.
4. Mix the Ingredients
   - Secure the spray top on the bottle and shake well to mix the ingredients thoroughly.
5. Label the Bottle

- o   Label the spray bottle with the date and the
    ingredients used for easy reference.
6. Use Your Spritzer

- o   Shake the bottle before each use to ensure the
    oils are evenly dispersed.
- o   Spray in the air, on linens, or directly onto your
    skin, avoiding sensitive areas like the eyes.
- o   For a calming effect, spray around your room or
    on your pillow before bed.
- o   For an invigorating boost, spray in the air
    around you or on your face (with eyes closed)
    during the day.

Tips for Creating Floraopathy™ Spritzers

- Quality Ingredients: Use high-quality, pure essential
  oils and distilled water or hydrosol to ensure the
  best therapeutic benefits.
- Patch Test: Before using the spritzer on your skin,
  perform a patch test to check for any sensitivity or
  allergic reactions.
- Storage: Store the spritzer in a cool, dark place to
  preserve the integrity of the essential oils.

By following these steps, you can create personalized
Floraopathy™ spritzers that cater to your specific needs and
preferences, enhancing your daily routine with the therapeutic
benefits of essential oils.

Miscellaneous Recipes

Bath Bomb Recipe

Ingredients:

1. 1 cup baking soda
2. 3/4 cup citric acid
3. 1/4 cup cornstarch
4. Approximately 20 drops of fragrant oil
5. 5-8 drops of soap colorant
6. Spritzer filled with water

Instructions:

1. Mix Dry Ingredients:
   - In a large mixing bowl, combine 1 cup of baking soda, 3/4 cup of citric acid, and 1/4 cup of cornstarch. Mix well to ensure all dry ingredients are thoroughly blended.
2. Add Fragrance:
   - While stirring the dry mixture, slowly add approximately 20 drops of fragrant oil. Continue to stir until the oil is evenly distributed throughout the mixture.
3. Add Colorant:
   - Add 5-8 drops of soap colorant to the mixture while stirring continuously. Ensure the color is evenly mixed in.
4. Add Water:
   - Begin to spritz the mixture with water while stirring constantly. The mixture should not look wet, so you'll need to check manually for the correct consistency.
   - Keep adding water by spraying more into the mixture while you stir. The goal is to achieve a

consistency that holds together when you squeeze it.

5. Check Consistency:
   - Periodically check the mixture by squeezing a handful. It should hold its shape and not crumble. If it's too dry, continue adding water a few spritzes at a time.

6. Fill Molds:
   - Once you have the correct consistency, fill your molds by packing the mixture down firmly. Ensure each mold is tightly packed to maintain the bath bomb's shape.

7. Turn Out Bath Bombs:
   - Prepare a baking sheet covered with parchment paper.
   - Cover each mold with the parchment paper and slowly turn it over to release the bath bomb. Carefully remove the plastic mold.

8. Drying:
   - Allow the bath bombs to dry overnight on the parchment paper. Once they are completely dry, they are ready to be packaged and used.

Tips:

1. Consistency Check: The key to a successful bath bomb is achieving the right consistency. It should feel like damp sand and hold together when squeezed.
2. Storage: Store the finished bath bombs in a cool, dry place to prevent them from absorbing moisture from the air.

Enjoy all the recipes: Aromatherapy Blending Tutorial with Dr. Constance Santego https://youtu.be/scVqiay_lUg

CHAPTER 8: INTEGRATING FLORAOPATHY™ WITH COMPLEMENTARY PRACTICES

Using Floraopathy™ with Other Vibrational Healing Practices

Floraopathy™ can be effectively integrated with various other vibrational healing practices to enhance its therapeutic benefits. Combining Floraopathy™ with complementary modalities can provide a holistic approach to healing, addressing the physical, emotional, mental, and spiritual aspects of well-being. Here are some key practices that synergize well with Floraopathy™:

1. Reiki

Overview: Reiki is a form of energy healing that involves the transfer of universal life energy through the practitioner's hands to the client. It balances the body's energy, promotes relaxation, and supports healing.

Integration with Floraopathy™:

> Reiki Sessions: Use Floraopathy™ blends during Reiki sessions to enhance energy flow and support healing.

Apply the blends topically or use a diffuser in the treatment room.

Chakra Balancing: Combine specific essential oil blends that resonate with each chakra to support energy alignment and balance.

2. Crystal Healing

Overview: Crystal healing uses the vibrational frequencies of crystals to balance the body's energy fields, promote healing, and enhance spiritual growth.

Integration with Floraopathy™:

Crystal Grids: Incorporate Floraopathy™ blends in crystal grids to amplify the energy and intention. Spritz the blends over the grid to infuse the crystals with the aromatic vibrations.

Meditation: Use essential oils that complement the properties of the crystals during meditation—for example, pair amethyst with lavender essential oil for relaxation and spiritual insight.

3. Sound Therapy

Overview: Sound therapy utilizes sound frequencies from instruments like singing bowls, tuning forks, and gongs to promote relaxation, release energy blockages, and support healing.

Integration with Floraopathy™:

Sound Baths: Diffuse Floraopathy™ blends in the room during sound baths to create a multi-sensory healing experience. The combination of sound and scent can deepen relaxation and enhance the therapeutic effects.

Personal Sessions: Apply essential oils to pulse points before sound therapy sessions to support energy flow and enhance the vibrational impact of the sound.

4. Aromatherapy

Overview: Aromatherapy is the use of essential oils for therapeutic purposes. It can be integrated with Floraopathy™ to enhance its physical, emotional, mental, and spiritual effects.

Integration with Floraopathy™:

Customized Blends: Create customized Floraopathy™ blends tailored to specific aromatherapy practices, such as inhalation, diffusion, or topical application.

Emotional Support: Use Floraopathy™ blends that target specific emotional issues during aromatherapy sessions to provide more profound emotional release and support.

5. Yoga and Meditation

Overview: Yoga and meditation are practices that promote physical flexibility, mental clarity, and spiritual growth. They are highly compatible with Floraopathy™.

Integration with Floraopathy™:

Yoga Practice: Diffuse essential oils in the yoga space or apply them topically before practice to enhance focus, relaxation, and energy flow.

Meditation: Use specific Floraopathy™ blends during meditation to support mental clarity, emotional balance, and spiritual connection.

6. Acupuncture and Traditional Chinese Medicine (TCM)

Overview: Acupuncture and TCM involve the use of needles, herbs, and other modalities to balance the body's energy (Qi) and promote healing.

Integration with Floraopathy™:

> Acupuncture Sessions: Apply Floraopathy™ blends to acupuncture points to enhance the flow of Qi and support the treatment.

> Herbal Remedies: Complement TCM herbal remedies with Floraopathy™ blends to provide a holistic approach to healing.

7. Reflexology

Overview: Reflexology involves applying pressure to specific points on the feet, hands, and ears that correspond to different body organs and systems.

Integration with Floraopathy™:

> Foot Reflexology: Use Floraopathy™ blends during reflexology sessions to enhance the therapeutic effects. Apply oils to the reflex points on the feet to support overall wellness.

> Hand Reflexology: Incorporate essential oils in hand reflexology sessions to provide additional relaxation and healing benefits.

Integrating Floraopathy™ with other vibrational healing practices creates a comprehensive and holistic approach to wellness. By combining the therapeutic properties of essential oils with complementary modalities, you can enhance the healing experience and support the body, mind, and spirit on a deeper level. This synergistic approach not only maximizes the benefits of each practice but also provides a more profound and enriching healing journey.

APPENDICES

Glossary of Terms for Floraopathy™

A

Aromatherapy: The practice of using essential oils extracted from plants for therapeutic purposes to enhance physical, emotional, and spiritual well-being.

Auric Massage: A technique that involves using essential oils to cleanse and balance the aura, the energy field surrounding the body.

B

Bath Bomb: A mixture of dry ingredients that effervesce when wet, used to add essential oils, scents, and other ingredients to bathwater for a therapeutic bathing experience.

Base Note: The longest-lasting scent in a blend, often derived from heavier oils that evaporate slowly, providing depth and grounding to the fragrance.

C

Carrier Oil: A vegetable oil derived from the fatty portion of a plant, such as the seeds, kernels, or nuts, used to dilute essential oils before topical application.

Chakra Balancing: The process of harmonizing the body's energy centers using various techniques, including the application of essential oils.

Crystal Healing: The use of crystals and gemstones to promote physical, emotional, and spiritual healing through their vibrational properties.

D

Diffuser: A device that disperses essential oils into the air, allowing for inhalation of their aromatic and therapeutic benefits.

Dilution: The process of reducing the concentration of essential oils by mixing them with a carrier oil or another medium to ensure safe application.

E

Essential Oil: A concentrated hydrophobic liquid containing volatile aroma compounds from plants, used in aromatherapy and Floraopathy™ for their therapeutic properties.

Edible Hydrosol: A hydrosol safe for consumption and used to flavor foods and beverages while providing subtle therapeutic benefits.

F

Floraopathy™: A unique approach to vibrational energy healing that utilizes the therapeutic properties of essential oils to create personalized treatments aimed at harmonizing the body, mind, and soul.

H

Hydrosol: The aromatic water that remains after steam distilling or hydrodistilling plant material, containing the water-soluble components of the plant.

I

Inhalation: The method of using essential oils by breathing them in, typically through a diffuser, steam, or direct inhalation.

J

Jacuzzi: A brand of hot tubs and whirlpool baths used here to refer to any hot tub in which essential oils can be used for inhalation benefits.

M

Master Blend: A concentrated mixture of essential oils used as a base for further dilutions in Floraopathy™ treatments.

Meditation: A practice where an individual uses techniques such as mindfulness, or focusing the mind on a particular object, thought, or activity to achieve a mentally clear and emotionally calm state.

Muscle Testing: A technique used to determine the body's response to various substances, including essential oils, by assessing muscle strength.

P

Planetary Healing: Using essential oils and other techniques in rituals to heal and balance the Earth's energies.

Potentization: The process of diluting and shaking a substance to enhance its energetic properties, often used in homeopathy and vibrational healing.

R

Reiki: A form of energy healing that involves the transfer of universal life energy through the practitioner's hands to the client, often enhanced by the use of essential oils.

S

Sauna (Wet): A steam room where essential oils can be used in the water to provide aromatic and therapeutic benefits through inhalation.

Sound Therapy: The use of sound frequencies from instruments like singing bowls, tuning forks, and gongs to promote relaxation, release energy blockages, and support healing.

Spritzer: A spray bottle used to disperse a mixture of essential oils and water or hydrosol for application to the skin or air.

Subtle Aromatherapy: The use of essential oils to affect the subtle body, psyche, and soul by drawing on their energetic or vibrational qualities.

T

Top Note: The initial scent in a blend that is perceived first but evaporates quickly, providing a fresh, uplifting aroma.

Therapeutic Cross Referencing (TCR): A method in Floraopathy™ for combining various therapeutic properties of essential oils to address multiple conditions simultaneously.

Traditional Chinese Medicine (TCM): A comprehensive medical system practiced for thousands of years, emphasizing the balance of Qi (vital energy) and the harmonious interaction of the Five Elements.

Y

Yoga: A group of physical, mental, and spiritual practices or disciplines that aim to control and still the mind, recognizing a detached witness-consciousness untouched by the mind (Chitta) and mundane suffering (Duḥkha).

FAQs on Using Floraopathy™ Blends

How often should a new blend be made?

The original blend is most effective for the first two months.

If the client does not achieve balance, create a new blend using a different combination of essential oils (ESOs).

Acute issues typically resolve within one to three months.

For chronic issues, expect it to take about one year for every ten years the issue has persisted to heal.

Will a client have any reactions?

Reactions are rare, but if a client is allergic to vodka, substitute with witch hazel or a vegetable solubilizer.

If you have checked all the client's contraindications, the blends should all be safe.

Can a client (adult or child) overdose?

No, clients cannot overdose on Floraopathy™ blends. The formulas work on a vibrational level and are best taken in small doses.

How Long Will Floraopathy™ Blends Last?

The shelf life of Floraopathy™ blends depends on several factors, including the type of essential oils used, the carrier oils, and the storage conditions. Following the same guidelines as aromatherapy and homeopathy, here's an overview of how long you can expect your Floraopathy™ blends to last:

Essential Oils Shelf Life

- Citrus Oils (e.g., lemon, orange, grapefruit): 6-12 months
- Most Essential Oils (e.g., lavender, peppermint, eucalyptus): 1-2 years
- Resin-Based Oils (e.g., frankincense, myrrh): 2-3 years
- Wood Oils (e.g., sandalwood, cedarwood): 2-4 years

Carrier Oils Shelf Life

- Jojoba Oil: 5 years (technically a wax, highly stable)
- Fractionated Coconut Oil: Indefinite (highly stable)
- Sweet Almond Oil: 1 year
- Olive Oil: 1-2 years
- Grapeseed Oil: 6-12 months

Blends Shelf-Life General Guidelines:

- Blends with Citrus Oils: 6-12 months
- Blends with Most Essential Oils: 1-2 years
- Blends with Resin-Based and Wood Oils: 2-3 years

Storage Tips

Dark Glass Bottles: Store blends in dark glass bottles to protect them from light exposure, which can degrade the oils.

Cool, Dark Place: Keep the bottles in a cool, dark place, away from direct sunlight and heat sources.

Tight Seals: Ensure that the bottles are tightly sealed to prevent oxidation and contamination.

Refrigeration: For longer shelf life, particularly for blends with citrus oils, consider storing them in the refrigerator.

By following these guidelines, you can maximize the shelf life and effectiveness of your Floraopathy™ blends, ensuring they remain potent and safe for use.

Sample Client Forms and Blending Charts

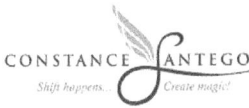

Holistic Healing Spa
Client Form

CONSTANCE ANTEGO
Shift happens...   Create magic!

PERSONAL INFORMATION

Name: Mr / Mrs / Ms / Miss _____ Birth Date: _____

Address: _____ City: _____

Phone: _____ Cell _____ Province: _____ Postal Code _____

E-Mail: _____ ONLY used for appointment reminders

YES ___, I would also like to be added to Connie's Health Tips & Tricks email list.

Occupation: _____ Hrs / Week ____ Work Activity: Sitting__ Standing __ Light labour __ Heavy labour __

Activities /Hobbies _____ Exercise _____ Steps / Day _____

Circle if Yes:

(only answer these if having Tinting, Facial or Back Treatment) - *ALL other treatments answer page three questions*

　　　Diabetes　Cancer　Epilepsy / Seizures　Arthritis　Aids　T.B.　Dermatitis　Hepatitis　Allergies _____

　　　Are you pregnant Y / N　　Any other Health Concerns we need to know about Y / N _____

How did you find us?

　　　Friend __ Mail __ Walk by __ Drive by__ Flyer __ Coupon __ Groupon __ Way Spa __ Other __

Client s Signature _____ Date: _____

Number the priority of these four -1being most important: Physical___ Mental___ Emotional ___ Spiritual ___

Quantum Healing___ Massage___ Reflexology___ Shiatsu___ Aromatherapy___ Tinting___ Facial___ Back Treatment___
Hypnotherapy___ Coaching___ (Goal setting_Releasing_), Reiki ___ Intuitive___ (Medium_ Tarot_ Angels_ Past Lives_)

WELLNESS INFORMATION

Most Important; What have you come for? _____

◆　Have you had this type of session before? Yes / No (If yes, when _____ and what type(s) _____).

◆　Pressure of the Massage; Do you like Light / Medium / Deep

Family Doctor: _____ Last Visit: _____
Chiropractor: ?　　　Physiotherapist:?　　　Massage Therapist:?　　　Other: ?

Surgeries:
Recent or past　No / Yes (if yes, please list below)
_____
_____

Injuries:
Recent or past　No / Yes (if yes, please list below)
_____
_____

CONTRA-INDICATIONS

Mark or Circled means: Ok or Checked ◆ *indicates mandatory questions*

go over these questions with your client and expand on anything they indicate they have or have had

◆ Muscular - Muscles — No / Yes _____
◆ Skeletal - Joints — No / Yes _____
◆ Digestive - Bowel — No / Yes _____
◆ Nerves CNS & PNS — No / Yes _____
◆ Skin — No / Yes _____
◆ Skin Rash — No / Yes _____
◆ Burns — No / Yes _____
◆ Cuts — No / Yes _____
◆ Bruises — No / Yes _____
Endocrine — No / Yes _____
Immune — No / Yes _____
Cold / Flu — No / Yes _____
Reproductive — No / Yes _____
◆ Pregnancy — No / Yes _____
Hysterectomy or Other — No / Yes _____
Menstruating — No / Yes _____
Vasectomy — No / Yes _____
Urinary - Bladder — No / Yes _____
◆ Lymph — No / Yes _____
◆ Respiratory — No / Yes _____
◆ Allergies — No / Yes _____
◆ Cardiovascular/Circulation — No / Yes _____
◆ Blood Pressure — H / L / N _____
◆ Heart Disease — No / Yes _____
◆ Varicose Veins — No / Yes _____
Inflammation — No / Yes _____
◆ Headaches — No / Yes _____
◆ Sleep (problems) — No / Yes _____
◆ Metal in the Body — No / Yes _____
◆ Energy — H / L / N _____
Vitamins — No / Yes _____
Medications — No / Yes _____
◆ Medications (affected by heat) — No / Yes _____
◆ Pain — No / Yes _____
Senses (eyes, ears, nose, touch, mouth) — No / Yes _____

Do you wear: Glasses contacts dentures hearing aids other_____

Circle if Yes: Diabetes Cancer Epilepsy / Seizures Arthritis Aids T.B. Dermatitis Hepatitis Other _____

COMMENTS: _____
_____
_____
_____
_____
_____

Therapy Used: please circle the following

Aromatherapy Reflexology - Foot or Hand Reiki / EB2 Table Shiatsu Iridology Muscle Testing (Kin) ELD Massage Hot Stone Massage
Swedish Massage Chair Massage Energy ECT Spa Other _____

Have you had or are you experiencing any issues of the following:

Soft Tissue (muscle)/Joint Discomfort	*Dizziness or Nausea*	Cancer Type _____
Arthritis (where) _____	*Allergies* _____	◊ Where _____
Osteoporosis _____	*Diabetes*	*Other Conditions*
Bone Fracture _____	*Head Aches* -how often _____	◊ Fibromyalgia / Chronic Fatigue
Numbness or Tingling		◊ Asthma / emphysema
Swelling / Inflammation / Stiffness	Sleep (Hrs. / Night___)	◊ Cerebral palsy
Front Back	Restful __ Restless __ Insomnia __	◊ Parkinson's
	Urinary / Bladder—Get up to go in night Y/N	◊ Nerves CNS / PNS
	Bowel Movements (# / day ___)	◊ Epilepsy / Seizures
	Skin	◊ MS
	◊ Skin Condition _____	◊ Endocrine _____
Pain today...	◊ Bruises or bruise easily	◊ Lymphatic
Where _____	◊ Cuts / Burns	◊ Other _____
Intensity Level (1 good -10 bad) _____	◊ Dermatitis	*Infections / Immune*
Neck	*Head / Neck*	◊ Cold / Flu / Fever
Shoulders	◊ Vision Problems / Vision Loss	◊ TB
Back: Lower, Mid, Upper	◊ Ear Problems / Aches / Hearing Loss	◊ Hepatitis
Arms	◊ Nose / Mouth	◊ HIV
Hands	*Cardiovascular*	◊ Other _____
Hips	◊ Varicose Veins / Stripped	*Women*
Legs	◊ Low __ High __ Blood pressure	◊ Birth Control
Knee	◊ CCHF	◊ Pregnant (Due date: _____)
Ankle or Feet	◊ Heart Attack	◊ # of Births _____
Metal In Body _____	◊ Phlebitis	◊ Menstruating / Hysterectomy / Menopause
Stress: Low __ Med __ High __	◊ Stroke / CVA	Other _____
Top Three (3) stressors	◊ Pacemaker or similar device	*Men* Vasectomy
_____	◊ Blood clots	Other _____
_____	◊ By Pass	*Respiratory*
_____	◊ Other	◊ Explain _____
_____	Radiation __ / Chemotherapy __	◊ Other
Energy Low__ Normal__ High__		

Medication / Vitamins No / Yes _____ Do you wear: Glasses Contacts Dentures Hearing aids Other _____
◆ Other Medical Conditions or Concerns _____

I have answered the questions above to the best of my ability. I acknowledge that massage therapy does not include a medical diagnosis. I authorize my practitioner to contact my medical doctor if need be. I give my consent for the massage session.

Client's Signature _____ Date. _____
Practitioner Findings: _____
_____
_____

Client Custom Blend	Student Case Study	Mark means OK

Client Acknowledgment and Permission: I acknowledge that;
- I have been informed about the Aromatherapy treatment being offered and I fully understand and accept this session is being performed by an Aromatherapist who is not a physician and can not diagnose or prescribe
- I am providing the information requested of my own free will and am not obliged in any way to do so. The information requested is to allow appropriate selection of oils and to ensure that a session is not contra-indicated
- I agree to this information being used as a part of the student aromatherapist's
- I do not wish this personal information shared with any other person or business, other than the instructor of the course

Name:_____ Address:_____

Phone:_____

Signature _____ Date _____

Contra-Indications

Blood Pressure	H / L / N	Aids	Y / N
Headaches	Y / N	Hepatitis	Y / N
Pregnancy	Y / N	Dermatitis	Y / N
Hyst / Other	Y / N	Insomnia	Y / N
Epilepsy / seizure:	Y / N	T.B.	Y / N
Allergies	Y / N		
Other (eg. Cancer)			

Circle and Number from 1 to 5 your main symptoms or conditions

Abdominal pain	Barber's rash	Congested skin	Endometriosis	Heartburn	Kidney infections	Orchitis	Skin disorders	Ulceration
Abscesses	Bed wetting	Congested lymph	Epilepsy	Heavy periods	Kidney - inflamed	Osteoporosis	Sore throat	Ulcers - gastric
Aches and Pains	Blood pressure	Constipation	Exhaustion	Hemorrhoids	Lactation	PMS	Spasticity	Vaginitis
Acne	Broken capillaries	Cough	Exposure	Hepatitis	Laryngitis	Periods - painful	Sports - performance	Varicose veins
Abdominal cramps	Bronchitis	Cramp	Fevers	Hernia	Leucorrhoea	Palpitations	Sprains	Varicocele
Abscess - dental	Bruises	Cuts / Abrasions	Fungal skin - warts	Hiccups	Lice	Paraplegia	Stings	Vomiting
Allergies - skin	Burns	Cystitis	Flatulence	High blood pressure	Liver problems	Parkinson's	Stomach ache	Warts
Allergies - general	Bursitis	Dandruff	Fluid retention	Hydrocele	Loss of appetite	Pleurisy	Stress	Whooping cough
Alopecia	Candida	Depression	Frigidity	Hysteria	Low blood pressure	Pneumonia	Sun burn	Writer's cramp
Alzheimer's	Carpal tunnel	Dermatitis	Ganglion	Impetigo	Lumbago	Prostatitis	Surgery	OF THE BODY
Amenorrhea	Catarrh	Diaper Rash	Gastro-enteritis	Impotence	Measles	Psoriasis	Swollen scrotum	SYSTEMS
Anti-aging	Cellulite	Diarrhea	Genital infection	Immune	Memory	Pyelitis	Swollen testicle	Genital / Urinary
Anxiety	Cerebral palsy	Digestion	Genital inflammation	Indigestion	Menopause	Respiratory fibrosit	Synovitis	Immune
Appetite (lack of)	Chapped lips/skin	Diverticulosis	Gout	Inflamed skin	Migraines	Rheumatism	Tendonitis	Lymph
Arthritis	Chicken pox	Dry / cracked skin	Gums - bleeding	Influenza	Mumps	Ring Worm	Tennis elbow	Reproductive
Asthma	Chilblains	Dysmenorrheal	Hangovers	Insect bites	Muscles	Scabies	Throat veins	Respiratory
Atheroma	Circulation	Ear ache	Hay fever	Insomnia	Muscular dystrophy	Scars	Throat infection	Skeletal
Arteriosclerosis	Cirrhosis	Ear infection	Headaches	Irregular periods	Nail infections	Sciatica	Thrush	Skin
Athlete's foot	Colds	Eczema	Heat rash	Irritable bowel	Nausea	Shingles	Tonsillitis	Mental
Back Pain	Cold sores	Edema	Heat stroke	Jet lag	Nervous	Shock	Torticollis	Muscles
Bal antic	Colic	Emotional Stress	Heart Care	Jock itch	Neuralgia	Sinus problems	Tuberculosis	Nerves

Main Condition			Secondary Condition			Third Condition		
STRESS								
TOP	MIDDLE	BASE	TOP	MIDDLE	BASE	TOP	MIDDLE	BASE
Bas	Cha	Ben						
Ber	Ger	C/W						
C/S	Hys	Fra						
Lem	Jun	Imm						
Man	Lav	Jas						
Ora	Mar	L/B						
Pet	Mel	Myr						
Thy	Pep	Ner						
Yar	Pin	Pat						
	R/M	Ros						
	R/W	S/w						
		Vet						
		Y/Y						

Oil	Oil	Oil	Oil	Carrier oil used		Cream ____	Lotion ____	Spritzer ____
						Oil ____	Other: ____	
# of drops	# of drops	# of drops	# of drops	5 % of other oil				

Acute / Chronic / Synergistic

Practitioner _____

Therapeutic Cross Reference Form

CLIENTS NAME: _____

Essential Oils Blend

Visit # _____   Signature _____   Date: _____

MAIN CONDITION			SECONDARY CONDITION		THIRD CONDITION	
	Stress					
Bas	Cha	Ben				
Ber	Ger	C/W				
C/S	Hys	Fra				
Lem	Jun	Imm				
Man	Lav	Jas				
Ora	Mar	L/B				
Pet	Mel	Myr				
Thy	Pep	Ner				
Yar	Pin	Pat				
	R/M	Ros				
	R/W	S/W				
		Vet				
		Y/Y				

Contra-Indications:

BLEND: Acute ____ Chronic ____ Synergistic ____   Cream ____ Lotion ____ Oil ____ Spritzer ____ Other _____

OIL -	OIL -	OIL -	OIL -	OIL -	Carrier Oil Used:	5% of the other Oil:
# of Drops ____	# of Drops ____	# of Drops ____	# of Drops ____	# of Drops ____	Crystals:	Herbs:

Visit # _____   Signature _____   Date: _____

MAIN CONDITION			SECONDARY CONDITION		THIRD CONDITION	
	Stress					
Bas	Cha	Ben				
Ber	Ger	C/W				
C/S	Hys	Fra				
Lem	Jun	Imm				
Man	Lav	Jas				
Ora	Mar	L/B				
Pet	Mel	Myr				
Thy	Pep	Ner				
Yar	Pin	Pat				
	R/M	Ros				
	R/W	S/W				
		Vet				
		Y/Y				

Contra-Indications:

BLEND: Acute ____ Chronic ____ Synergistic ____   Cream ____ Lotion ____ Oil ____ Spritzer ____ Other _____

OIL -	OIL -	OIL -	OIL -	OIL -	Carrier Oil Used:	5% of the other Oil:
# of Drops ____	# of Drops ____	# of Drops ____	# of Drops ____	# of Drops ____	Crystals:	Herbs:

Practitioner _____

Essential Oil Stores

Floraopathy™ is founded on the principles of Therapeutic Cross Referencing (TCR) principles and suggests high-quality essential oils from New Directions Aromatics.

New Directions Aromatics

Website: https://www.newdirectionsaromatics.com/

> New Directions Aromatics operates globally, with companies located in various countries. When purchasing from their website, ensure you are selecting the correct country to source your products.

Description: New Directions Aromatics (NDA) is a leading supplier of wholesale essential oils, carrier oils, and other natural products. They serve a wide range of industries, including aromatherapy, personal care, and cosmetics. NDA is known for its extensive product range, high quality, and competitive prices.

Key Features of New Directions Aromatics

1. Extensive Product Range:
   - Essential Oils: NDA offers a vast selection of essential oils, including popular choices like lavender, peppermint, and tea tree, as well as more exotic options.
   - Carrier Oils: A wide variety of carrier oils, such as jojoba, sweet almond, and argan oil, are available for diluting essential oils and making custom blends.
   - Hydrosols: NDA provides a range of hydrosols (floral waters) for use in skincare and aromatherapy.

- Butters and Waxes: High-quality natural butters and waxes, including shea butter and beeswax, are offered for making lotions, balms, and other personal care products.
- Clays and Salts: Various clays and salts are available for use in bath and body products.

2. Quality Assurance:
   - GC-MS Testing: NDA conducts Gas Chromatography-Mass Spectrometry (GC-MS) testing on their essential oils to ensure purity and quality. These reports are available upon request.
   - Organic and Conventional Options: They offer both organic and conventional essential oils, catering to different customer needs.

3. Sustainability and Ethical Sourcing:
   - Ethical Sourcing: NDA is committed to sourcing its products ethically and working with suppliers who practice sustainable farming and harvesting methods.
   - Sustainability Initiatives: They emphasize environmental responsibility and sustainability in their business practices.

4. Wholesale Pricing:
   - Competitive Prices: NDA offers competitive wholesale pricing, making it an excellent choice for businesses and practitioners looking to purchase essential oils and natural products in bulk.
   - No Minimum Order: They do not require a minimum order, allowing customers to purchase the quantities they need.

5. Educational Resources:
   - Product Information: Detailed product descriptions, including the botanical name,

extraction method, and country of origin, are provided for each item.
- o Usage Guidelines: NDA offers guidelines on how to use their products safely and effectively in various applications.

Companies Selling Food-Grade Essential Oils

1. Young Living

Website: https://www.youngliving.com/

Description: Young Living offers a line of essential oils called Vitality™, which are specifically labeled for dietary use. These oils are safe for culinary applications and are rigorously tested for quality and purity.

2. doTERRA

Website: https://www.doterra.com/

Description: doTERRA's essential oils labeled as "Certified Pure Therapeutic Grade®" (CPTG) include a line of oils that are safe for internal use. Their culinary collection is designed for use in cooking and beverages.

3. Plant Therapy

Website: https://www.planttherapy.com/

Description: Plant Therapy offers a range of USDA organic essential oils that are labeled for food and dietary use. They provide detailed information on which oils are safe to ingest.

4. Eden's Garden

Website: https://www.edensgarden.com/

Description: Eden's Garden provides a selection of essential oils that are labeled as GRAS (Generally Recognized As Safe) by the FDA for food use. They emphasize purity and quality testing.

5. Mountain Rose Herbs

Website: https://www.mountainroseherbs.com/

Description: Mountain Rose Herbs offers a variety of organic essential oils that are safe for culinary use. They provide detailed product descriptions and usage guidelines.

6. Now Foods

Website: https://www.nowfoods.com/

Description: NOW Foods offers a line of essential oils that are safe for culinary applications. Their oils are rigorously tested for purity and quality.

7. Aura Cacia

Website: https://www.auracacia.com/

Description: Aura Cacia provides essential oils that are suitable for food use. They offer detailed guidelines on how to safely use their oils in cooking and beverages.

8. Rocky Mountain Oils

> Website: https://www.rockymountainoils.com/

> Description: Rocky Mountain Oils offers a selection of essential oils that are safe for internal use. They provide information on the purity and safety of their products.

9. Simply Earth

> Website: https://simplyearth.com/

> Description: Simply Earth provides essential oils that are safe for ingestion and culinary use. They focus on providing pure and high-quality oils at affordable prices.

Safety Considerations

- Dilution: Always dilute essential oils properly before ingesting them. Typically, one drop of essential oil is sufficient for flavoring a large quantity of food or drink.
- Purity: Ensure that the essential oils are labeled as food-grade or safe for internal use. Not all essential oils are suitable for ingestion.
- Consultation: If you are unsure about the safety of ingesting a particular essential oil, consult with a healthcare provider or a certified aromatherapist.

Do your homework and research the company before purchasing any products. By choosing high-quality, food-grade essential oils from reputable companies, you can safely incorporate the therapeutic and flavor benefits of essential oils into your culinary creations.

Companies Selling Aromatherapy Bottles

1. New Directions Aromatics

    Website: https://www.newdirectionsaromatics.com/

    Description: Offers a wide range of packaging options, including glass bottles, plastic bottles, jars, and closures suitable for essential oils and aromatherapy products.

2. SKS Bottle & Packaging

    Website: https://www.sks-bottle.com/

    Description: Provides a comprehensive selection of glass and plastic bottles, jars, tins, and closures. They cater to the needs of the aromatherapy and personal care industries.

3. Specialty Bottle

    Website: https://www.specialtybottle.com/

    Description: Offers high-quality glass and plastic bottles, jars, and tins at wholesale prices. They have a variety of styles and sizes ideal for essential oils and aromatherapy products.

4. Bulk Apothecary

    Website: https://www.bulkapothecary.com/

    Description: Supplies a wide range of packaging solutions, including glass bottles, plastic bottles, jars, and caps. They are a popular choice for packaging for essential oil and aromatherapy products.

5. Glassnow

   Website: https://www.glassnow.com/

   Description: Focuses on eco-friendly glass packaging, offering bottles and jars made from recycled glass. They provide various styles suitable for aromatherapy and essential oils.

6. Berlin Packaging

   Website: https://www.berlinpackaging.com/

   Description: A major supplier of packaging products, including glass and plastic bottles, jars, and closures. They offer customizable options for the aromatherapy industry.

7. Uline

   Website: https://www.uline.com/

   Description: Provides a wide selection of packaging supplies, including bottles and jars for essential oils and aromatherapy products. They offer bulk purchasing options.

8. Elements Bath & Body

   Website: https://www.elementsbathandbody.com/

   Description: Specializes in packaging and supplies for personal care and aromatherapy products, including a variety of bottles, jars, and tins.

9. Sunburst Bottle

Website: https://www.sunburstbottle.com/

Description: Offers a variety of glass and plastic bottles and jars suitable for essential oils, with various closures and accessories.

10. Got Oil Supplies

Website: https://www.gotoilsupplies.com/

Description: Specializes in essential oil supplies, including a wide range of bottles, roller bottles, sprayers, and other accessories for aromatherapy enthusiasts and professionals.

Considerations When Purchasing Aromatherapy Bottles

- Material: Choose between glass and plastic based on your needs. Glass is generally preferred for essential oils due to its non-reactive properties.
- Size: Consider the sizes you need, from small sample vials to larger bottles for blends and storage.
- Closure Type: Look for secure closures such as droppers, spray tops, roller tops, or screw caps, depending on your intended use.
- Quality: Ensure the bottles are of high quality and suitable for storing essential oils without degradation.

Bulk Options: If you need a large quantity, look for companies that offer bulk purchasing at competitive prices.

By selecting a reputable supplier, you can ensure that your aromatherapy bottles meet the quality and functionality standards necessary for storing and using essential oils effectively.

Recommended Reading and Resources for Floraopathy™

Books

1. **"Secrets of a Healer, Magic of Aromatherapy" by Dr. Constance Santego**
   o The complete manual is for the Standard Aromatherapy Course.
2. **"Secrets of a Healer, Magic of Muscle Testing" by Dr. Constance Santego**
   o The complete manual to Muscle Testing Course.
3. **"The Complete Guide to Aromatherapy" by Salvatore Battaglia**
   o A comprehensive resource covering the principles and practices of aromatherapy, including the therapeutic use of essential oils.
4. **"Aromatherapy for Healing the Spirit" by Gabriel Mojay**
   o Explores the use of essential oils in the context of traditional Chinese medicine and its applications for emotional and spiritual healing.
5. **"The Encyclopedia of Essential Oils" by Julia Lawless**
   o An extensive reference guide detailing the properties, uses, and applications of over 160 essential oils.
6. **"Essential Oil Safety: A Guide for Health Care Professionals" by Robert Tisserand and Rodney Young**
   o An authoritative source on the safety and toxicology of essential oils, providing detailed information on safe usage practices.
7. **"Advanced Aromatherapy: The Science of Essential Oil Therapy" by Kurt Schnaubelt**

- o Delves into the scientific basis of essential oil therapy and its practical applications in health and wellness.

8. **"Hydrosols: The Next Aromatherapy" by Suzanne Catty**
   - o Focuses on the therapeutic use of hydrosols, the aromatic water solutions obtained from steam distillation of plants.

9. **"Aromatherapy for Common Ailments" by Shirley Price**
   - o Offers practical advice and recipes for using essential oils to address a wide range of common health issues.

10. **"The Complete Book of Essential Oils and Aromatherapy" by Valerie Ann Worwood**
    - o A versatile guide that includes over 800 recipes for health, beauty, and home care using essential oils.

11. **"The Art of Herbal Healing: Herbalism for Beginners" by Ava Green**
    - o Introduces the basics of herbal medicine and the integration of essential oils and herbs in holistic healing practices.

12. **"Essential Oils for Emotional Wellbeing: More Than 400 Recipes for Mind, Emotions, and Spirit" by Vannoy Gentles Fite**
    - o Provides recipes and guidance on using essential oils to support emotional health and spiritual well-being.

Online Resources

National Association for Holistic Aromatherapy (NAHA)

> Website: https://naha.org/

> Offers educational resources, certification programs, and articles on aromatherapy practices and essential oil safety.

Alliance of International Aromatherapists (AIA)

> Website: https://www.alliance-aromatherapists.org/

> Provides information on aromatherapy education, conferences, and research.

Tisserand Institute

> Website: https://tisserandinstitute.org/

> Focuses on essential oil safety, providing research articles, webinars, and educational courses.

AromaWeb

> Website: https://www.aromaweb.com/

> A comprehensive resource offering essential oil profiles, recipes, and articles on aromatherapy.

Plant Therapy Blog

> Website: https://www.planttherapy.com/blog/

> Provides articles, guides, and DIY recipes related to essential oils and their uses.

New Directions Aromatics Blog

> Website:
> https://www.newdirectionsaromatics.com/blog/

> Features articles on essential oil profiles, benefits, and applications in personal care and aromatherapy.

Edens Garden Blog

> Website: https://www.edensgarden.com/blogs/news

> Offers educational content, DIY recipes, and tips for using essential oils safely and effectively.

Revive Essential Oils Blog

> Website: https://www.revive-eo.com/blogs/news

> Provides insights, guides, and practical uses for essential oils in everyday life.

Courses and Workshops

1. Dr. Constance Santego's Courses are offered through 3Jinn Business Hub.
   - Floraopathy™
   - Muscle Testing
   - Website: https://3jinn.com/floraopathy-certificate-course/
2. Aromahead Institute
   - Website: https://www.aromahead.com/
   - Offers comprehensive online courses in aromatherapy, essential oil safety, and blending techniques.
3. School for Aromatic Studies
   - Website: https://aromaticstudies.com/

- o Provides online and in-person courses on aromatherapy, natural perfumery, and herbalism.
4. Tisserand Institute Courses
   - o Website: https://tisserandinstitute.org/education/
   - o Offers online courses focused on essential oil safety, advanced aromatherapy, and blending.
5. International School of Aromatherapy
   - o Website: https://www.isoa.org/
   - o Provides certification programs and workshops in aromatherapy and essential oil applications.
6. Floracopeia Essential Oils and Aromatherapy Courses
   - o Website: https://www.floracopeia.com/
   - o Offers educational resources and online courses on essential oils, herbalism, and natural health.

These recommended readings and resources will provide a solid foundation in the principles and practices of Floraopathy™, enhancing your understanding and application of essential oils and vibrational healing.

BIBLIOGRAPHY

Dr. Constance's YouTube Videos: AROMATHERAPY (10+ videos)
Blending   https://youtu.be/scVqiay_lUg

Books and Articles

1. **Santego, Dr. Constance.** *Secrets of a Healer, Magic of Aromatherapy,* 2020.
   - The complete manual is for the Standard Aromatherapy Course.
2. **Battaglia, Salvatore.** *The Complete Guide to Aromatherapy.* The International Centre of Holistic Aromatherapy, 2003.
   - A comprehensive guide covering the principles and practices of aromatherapy.
3. **Davis, Patricia.** *Aromatherapy: An A-Z.* Vermilion, 2005.
   - An alphabetical guide to essential oils and their therapeutic uses.
4. **Lavabre, Marcel.** *Aromatherapy Workbook.* Healing Arts Press, 1997.
   - A practical guide to the therapeutic applications of essential oils.
5. **Price, Shirley, and Len Price.** *Aromatherapy for Health Professionals.* Churchill Livingstone, 2011.
   - A detailed textbook for health professionals on the clinical use of essential oils.

6. **Rose, Jeanne.** *375 Essential Oils and Hydrosols.* Frog Ltd, 1999.
    - A comprehensive reference for essential oils and hydrosols, including their properties and uses.
7. **Schnaubelt, Kurt.** *Advanced Aromatherapy: The Science of Essential Oil Therapy.* Healing Arts Press, 1998.
    - An in-depth look at the scientific basis of essential oil therapy.
8. **Tisserand, Robert, and Rodney Young.** *Essential Oil Safety: A Guide for Health Care Professionals.* Churchill Livingstone, 2013.
    - A crucial resource on the safety considerations and toxicology of essential oils.
9. **Worwood, Valerie Ann.** *The Complete Book of Essential Oils and Aromatherapy.* New World Library, 2016.
    - An extensive guide on the uses and benefits of essential oils in everyday life.

Research Papers and Journals

9. **Buchbauer, G., Jirovetz, L., Jager, W., Plank, C., & Dietrich, H.** "Fragrance Compounds and Essential Oils with Sedative Effects upon Inhalation." *Journal of Pharmaceutical Sciences*, 82(6), 1993, pp. 660-664.
    - Research on the sedative effects of certain essential oils when inhaled.
10. **Fowler, N. A.** "Aromatherapy and Cancer Care: A Review of the Literature." *International Journal of Palliative Nursing*, 9(9), 2003, pp. 444-448.
    - A review of the application of aromatherapy in cancer care settings.
11. **Hart, S., & Board, R.** "Complementary Therapies in Nursing Practice: Aromatherapy." *Nursing Standard*, 15(15), 2001, pp. 33-38.

o   A discussion on the integration of aromatherapy in nursing practice.

12. **Perry, N., & Perry, E.** "Aromatherapy in the Management of Psychiatric Disorders: Clinical and Neuropharmacological Perspectives." *Central Nervous System Agents in Medicinal Chemistry*, 6(4), 2006, pp. 279-287.

o   An exploration of the use of aromatherapy in treating psychiatric disorders.

Websites and Online Resources

13. **National Association for Holistic Aromatherapy (NAHA).** *Aromatherapy.* Retrieved from https://naha.org/

o   A resource for education and information on aromatherapy practices.

14. **Aromatherapy Science Blog.** "The Benefits and Uses of Hydrosols." Retrieved from https://aromatherapysciences.blogspot.com/

o   An informative blog on the various uses of hydrosols in aromatherapy.

15. **Tisserand Institute.** "Essential Oil Safety." Retrieved from https://tisserandinstitute.org/

o   A comprehensive resource on the safety and proper use of essential oils.

Aromatherapy Associations around the Globe

Canada

1. **Canadian Federation of Aromatherapists (CFA)**

o   **Website**: https://cfacanada.com/

o   **Description**: The CFA is dedicated to advancing the practice of aromatherapy in Canada. They offer certification programs, professional development, and support for aromatherapists.

2. **British Columbia Alliance of Aromatherapy (BCAOA)**
   - **Website:** https://bcaoa.org/
   - **Description:** BCAOA provides education, certification, and support to aromatherapists in British Columbia. They focus on maintaining high standards of practice and promoting public awareness of aromatherapy.

3. **Ontario Aromatherapy Association (OAA)**
   - **Website:** http://ontarioaromatherapy.ca/
   - **Description:** OAA offers resources, training, and certification for aromatherapists in Ontario. They aim to enhance the credibility and professional standards of aromatherapy.

USA

1. **National Association for Holistic Aromatherapy (NAHA)**
   - **Website:** https://naha.org/
   - **Description:** NAHA is a leading organization in the USA dedicated to holistic aromatherapy education and practice. They provide certification programs, resources, and professional networking opportunities for aromatherapists.

2. **Alliance of International Aromatherapists (AIA)**
   - **Website:** https://www.alliance-aromatherapists.org/
   - **Description:** AIA promotes the scientific and educational aspects of aromatherapy. They offer certification, conferences, and resources for professional development in the field.

3. **Aromatherapy Registration Council (ARC)**
   - **Website**: https://aromatherapycouncil.org/
   - **Description**: ARC provides the Registered Aromatherapist (RA) credential, setting high standards for professional aromatherapy practice. They aim to ensure the competency and ethical practice of aromatherapists.

International

1. **International Federation of Aromatherapists (IFA)**
   - **Website**: https://ifaroma.org/
   - **Description**: The IFA is a global organization that sets high standards for aromatherapy education and practice. They offer certification, professional development, and resources for aromatherapists worldwide.
2. **International Aromatherapy and Aromatic Medicine Association (IAAMA)**
   - **Website**: https://iaama.org.au/
   - **Description**: Based in Australia, IAAMA promotes the professional practice of aromatherapy and aromatic medicine. They provide accreditation, education, and support for practitioners globally.
3. **International Alliance of Professional Aromatherapists (IAPA)**
   - **Website**: http://iapaglobal.com/
   - **Description**: IAPA aims to unify professional aromatherapists around the world, offering resources, education, and a platform for sharing knowledge and best practices.

Europe

1. **Aromatherapy Trade Council (ATC)**
   - o **Website**: https://www.a-t-c.org.uk/
   - o **Description**: The ATC represents the interests of the aromatherapy industry in the UK and Europe, promoting high standards of practice and safety in the production and use of essential oils.
2. **European Federation of Essential Oils (EFEO)**
   - o **Website**: https://www.efeo.org/
   - o **Description**: EFEO is dedicated to ensuring the quality and safety of essential oils within Europe. They provide guidelines, advocacy, and support for industry professionals.

Asia-Pacific

1. **Asia-Pacific Aromatherapy Association (APAA)**
   - o **Website**: http://apaa.org.au/
   - o **Description**: The APAA supports the aromatherapy profession in the Asia-Pacific region, offering education, certification, and resources for practitioners.
2. **Japan Aromatherapy Association (JAA)**
   - o **Website**: https://www.jaa-aroma.or.jp/
   - o **Description**: JAA promotes the safe and effective use of aromatherapy in Japan. They offer certification programs, educational resources, and professional development for aromatherapists.

Africa

1. **South African Association of Aromatherapists (SAAH)**
   - o **Website**: http://www.saah.co.za/
   - o **Description**: SAAH supports the practice of aromatherapy in South Africa, providing education, certification, and resources for practitioners.

South America

1. **Brazilian Association of Aromatherapy and Aromatic Medicine (ABRAROMA)**
   - o **Website**: http://abraroma.org.br/
   - o **Description**: ABRAROMA promotes the practice of aromatherapy and aromatic medicine in Brazil, offering education, certification, and professional development.

These associations offer valuable resources, certification programs, and support for aromatherapists, promoting the professional practice and education of aromatherapy.

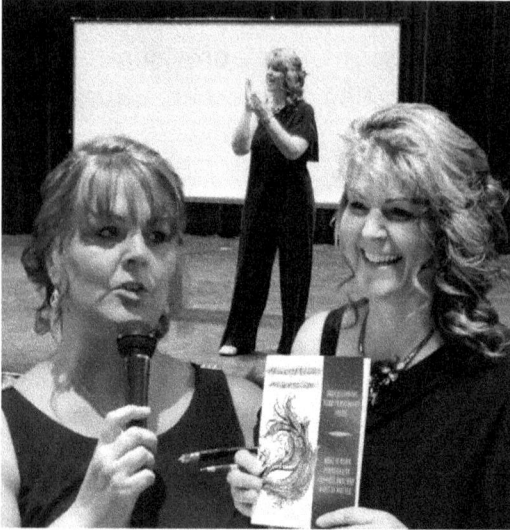

Dr. Constance Santego: A Pioneer in Holistic Health and Floraopathy™

Dr. Constance Santego: A Pioneer in Holistic Health and Floraopathy™

Dr. Constance Santego is a distinguished expert in holistic health and spiritual healing, with over twenty-five years of experience teaching these subjects. She possesses a profound understanding of the interconnectedness of the mind, body, and spirit in achieving overall well-being.

Dr. Santego holds a Ph.D. and a Doctorate in Natural Medicine, providing her with an in-depth knowledge of alternative healing modalities and their application in promoting optimal health. Her extensive educational background enables her to address health concerns from a holistic perspective, considering the physical, emotional, and spiritual aspects of an individual's well-being.

Throughout her career, Dr. Santego has been dedicated to sharing her knowledge and empowering others to take control of their health and healing. She uniquely blends scientific research and traditional wisdom, creating a bridge between conventional and alternative medicine.

In addition to her expertise in various holistic practices, Dr. Santego is proficient in Aromatherapy and Floraopathy™. Her innovative approach combines the ancient wisdom of essential oils and their healing properties with modern techniques to create customized blends for individual health concerns. Through extensive research and practical application, Dr. Santego has developed a system that helps individuals achieve balance and well-being by using specific essential oil blends tailored to their unique needs.

Dr. Santego also contributes her extensive knowledge through her "Secrets of a Healer" educational series. Drawing upon her vast experience and expertise, she captivates readers with her insights and teachings. She takes readers on a transformative journey, delving into the realms of holistic health, spirituality, and self-discovery. Through her writing, she aims to inspire individuals to tap into their innate healing abilities and embrace a balanced and harmonious approach to well-being.

Her work has profoundly impacted many, guiding them toward a deeper understanding of themselves and their connection to the world around them. Her series serves as a beacon of wisdom, offering practical tools and techniques for personal growth and transformation.

Dr. Constance Santego's unique blend of knowledge, experience, and passion makes her a captivating figure in holistic health, spiritual healing, and Aromatherapy and Floraopathy™. Her contributions through teaching, writing, and her spellbinding series continue to inspire and empower individuals on their journeys toward well-being and self-discovery.

Message from the Author, Dr. Constance Santego

Welcome to the transformative world of Floraopathy™. This book is designed to provide you with an overview of the art and science of essential oils, setting the foundation for your journey of self-discovery and healing. The techniques shared here are rooted in ancient wisdom and enhanced by modern holistic practices, empowering you to take control of your health and well-being.

To fully harness the power of Floraopathy™ and perform sessions effectively, I encourage you to take the comprehensive Floraopathy™ course. This course delves deeper into the methods outlined in this book, offering detailed instructions, hands-on training, and the certification required to practice Floraopathy™ professionally. By becoming certified, you will be equipped to provide personalized and effective healing sessions for yourself and others.

Explore the methods in this book, and let them inspire you to further your knowledge through the Floraopathy™ course. Trust in your ability to connect with the vibrational energy of plants and make informed decisions about your health. The journey to becoming a certified practitioner will enhance your skills and understanding, allowing you to offer transformative healing to those around you.

Embark on this journey to well-being and professional growth through the power of Floraopathy™!

Warm regards, Dr. Constance Santego

ALSO AVAILABLE

Ring Therapy Practitioner Certification Program

The Ring Therapy Practitioner Certification Program is a comprehensive course designed for individuals seeking to master the art of ring therapy for holistic healing. This program delves into the principles of Traditional Chinese Medicine (TCM), Ayurveda, and modern holistic practices, teaching you how to use metal rings to balance and enhance various body systems. You'll learn to apply these techniques effectively through detailed modules and hands-on practicum, providing personalized health solutions. Join us to gain valuable skills and become a certified practitioner, ready to help others achieve optimal health and well-being through ring therapy.

READ MORE:

https://constancesantego.ca/ring-therapy/

https://3jinn.com/courses/ring-therapy-practitioner-certification-program/

Go to our website to sign up and receive "Email Notifications" for upcoming Seminars, APPs, and other relevant information.

PLAY THE GAME *IKONA* – DISCOVER YOUR INNER GENIE

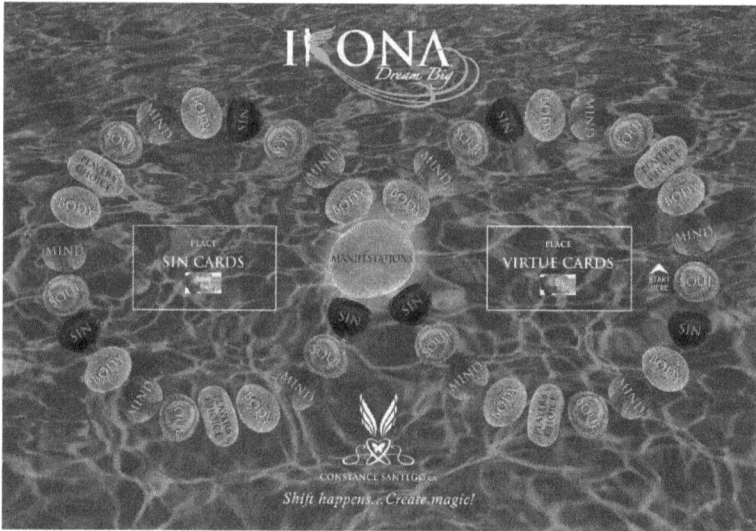

For additional information on

Constance Santego's

wide range of Motivational Products, Coaching Sessions,
Spiritual Retreats,
Live Events and Educational Programs

Go to

www.ConstanceSantego.ca

Follow on Instagram - Constance_Santego and
Facebook - constancesantegoo

Subscribe and receive Free Information and Meditations on my
YouTube Channel - Constance Santego

www.ingramcontent.com/pod-product-compliance
Lightning Source LLC
Chambersburg PA
CBHW060235030426
42335CB00014B/1474